Endorsements for
"Darwin's Replacement" (First Edition)

"The need for a superintelligent force to create and sustain living things is well set out and without question. I also appreciated all the research that was done to demonstrate the historical importance and recognition of God in the nation lives of the four nations you selected."   -- George Matzko, PhD

"*Darwin's Replacement* is a well-written review of the enormous complexity of all life from the perspective of the molecular foundation. The complexity is more than amazing. Most people enjoy learning about amazing feats, and thus the popularity of 'Ripley's Believe It or Not' and similar books. Our body and its complexity is familiar to all and works so well for most of us that we often take it for granted. Mr. Rogers' book helps us to realize that we are all walking miracles and understanding how it functions is both awe-inspiring and helps us to appreciate the body we all live in while on this earth."

-- Jerry Bergman, PhD

"*Darwin's Replacement* provides a credible assessment of the weaknesses within mainstream evolution theory and proposes a reasonable, evidence-based alternative for the origin and development of life."   -- Nicholas Comninellis, MD MPH

"ATOMIC BIOLOGY promises to restore the true foundations of science back to the realm of observation. Current forays into metaphysical speculation and presupposition by 'experts' seem to have caused division, confusion, and misunderstanding in the scientific conversation."   -- Jack Taylor, PhD

"My recommendation would be to rework the book as a series of 1-2 page studies for adult Sunday school classes and/or Christian High School classes. It could be useful as an introduction to the topics, in that format."   -- David Snoke, PhD

"Your book demonstrates the amazing complexity of life, starting with even the simplest cell, and the numerous conditions needed to sustain life. That all this could be the result of blind, random evolution is highly implausible, and statistically virtually impossible. Hence, as your book concludes, this points to a superintelligent Creator. Your book also notes that the USA, the UK, Canada, and Australia were all founded on submission to the Christian God, and urges those countries return to acknowledging God, also in science classrooms.

I heartily agree with all this."   -- John Byl, PhD

"There are only two possibilities for the existence of life: accidental or purposeful. Using science and mathematics, Atomic Biology proves beyond a shadow of doubt that life cannot be accidental. Then the book shows that the only being capable of the creation of life and its orchestrated maintenance is the historical Omniscient, Omnipotent, and Omnipresent Triune God of the Bible and our Nation."   -- Sharon E. Cargo, DVM

"Hi, (LRG): I recently bought the book and am reading it slowly and out loud to myself so that it sticks, but can I say that when I heard Mr. Rogers on Vision I knew that this was a book I'd been waiting for a very long time. I honestly can't put into words how exciting this is for me to finally have something I can refer to when discussing creation and not sound like a loony."
                          -- Linda Houston, Australia

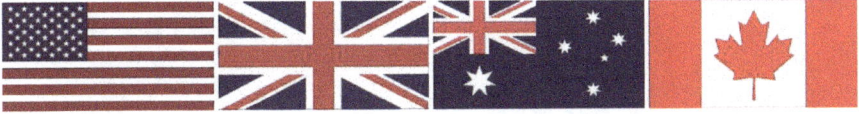

Flags of Four of the Nations Where God Is Part of Government   *

DARWIN'S REPLACEMENT SERIES - TEXTBOOK

"GOD'S BIOLOGY"
DARWIN'S REPLACEMENT

JERRY BERGMAN - GRAHAM McLENNAN – THOMAS ROGERS

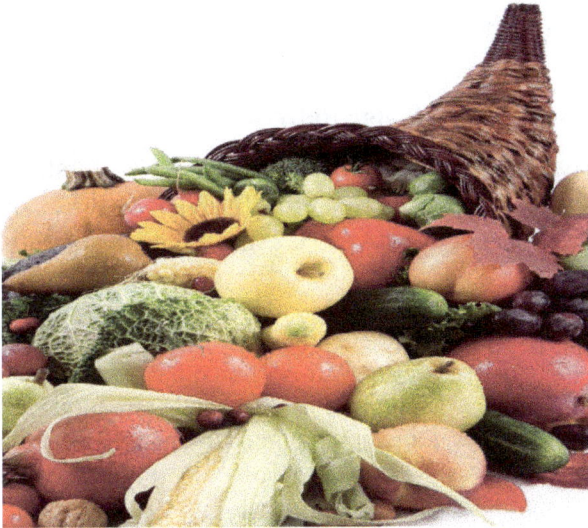

Olga Lyubkina/Shutterstock.com

How are we so amazingly made and cared for? Research now shows us that it requires a superintelligent, reliable, and caring being. Our Governments and the majority of our citizens call this being, "God." He makes us from the "dust" using His awesome two-step process: (1) selecting the correct atoms from the soil to create our grown foods, then (2) selecting the correct atoms from our foods to create our cell parts and us.

Who else can make our grown foods and us out of "dust"?

*Shutterstock Flags: US & UK - Claudio Divisia; Aus.- Artgraphixel; Can. – Jannoon028

DARWIN'S REPLACEMENT SERIES – TEXTBOOK

"GOD'S BIOLOGY"
DARWIN'S REPLACEMENT

Part of "THE TRUTH FOR LIFE EDUCATION PROJECT"

LRG

LIFETIME REFERENCE GUIDES INC.
P.O.Box 51613 RPO Park Royal
West Vancouver, BC, Canada   V7T 2X9

www.lifetimereferenceguides.com

ISBNs
978-1-9992097-9-7   (Hardcover)
978-1-7383082-0-0   (Paperback)
978-1-7383082-1-7   (eBook)

Science
Life
Education
Government

Contents

Dedication

To our superintelligent and caring Creator, credit for all Life where all credit is due.

Regardless of our race, color, belief, or creed, He makes all our grown foods from dust and all our amazing parts from these foods.

No one else has this ability, cares this much, or works this hard for each one of us every second of every day.

This is why He is so highly recognized by our governments and by so many citizens as our Creator, God, Whom we can trust.

Acknowledgements

Our respect and gratitude go to the forty-five scholars whose work has helped in the discovery and development of this God-based life science called "Atomic Biology" and nicknamed "God's Biology."

Our Creator has probably been using this science since the beginning along with all His other sciences.

We are especially grateful to Dr. Gerald Bergman, PhD, Dr. Graham McLennan, DDS, Bonnie Rogers, RN, BScN, editor David V. Bassett, MSc, and director Norman Wright, for their significant input.

Our gratitude also goes to the many contributors, encouragers, and endorsers who have helped to keep this work moving forward.

Tom Rogers, President
The Atomic Biology Institute

INTRODUCTION

The central focus of this book and science is verifying this: "WITHOUT THE TRIUNE GOD OF OUR WESTERN NATIONS, THERE WOULD BE NO FOOD AND NO LIFE."

First, let's clear away two common stumbling blocks:

(1) For those who think we cannot teach publicly about our Creator, God, because of the (mis)conception regarding "Separation of church and state." Please understand why God is NOT "the church." "Churches" are buildings or groups of people who may be Satanists, New Agers, Catholics, Protestants, Mormons, Jehovah's Witnesses, or hundreds of cults. No church can create any living entity. So "God" is definitely NOT "the church."

God is highly respected for several clear and solid reasons by many churches, just as He is highly respected by our national governments, as in "One Nation Under God," "In God We Trust," (and more in USA), "God Save The King," (and more in UK), "Whereas Canada is founded on principles that recognize the Supremacy of God...," (and more in Canada), in Australia's constitution, "... humbly relying on the blessing of Almighty God," (and more in Australia). (See Chapters 10-13).

(2) Be aware of the most influential troublemaker on Planet Earth, Public Enemy #1, Satan himself, with his many (perhaps unaware) atheistic followers who are determined to remove God from our society. They would starve to death if not fed by God.

This book is written to provide some beneficial Truths For Life that have been missing from our public education system. Teachers and professors have been forced to teach information about Life that many of them disagree with, but currently, they cannot change. Basically, the teaching that is enforced at this time is that life 'arose' by a chance arrangement of molecules to make a reproducing cell called a "common ancestor." From this theoretical cell 'came' more complex cells which gradually gave birth to all life in the world with no guidance, no intelligence, and definitely no God. That is what is being legally taught throughout virtually all public education in the Western world. Teachers and professors have to teach this even in many Christian institutions.

INTRODUCTION

This book focuses on the *true* origin and cause of Life.

Have you ever thought of all the amazing and careful works our Creator performs for each one of us every second of every day?

If not, you are certainly not alone, and for some understandable reasons. Because His works are so constant and reliable, like making our foods out of dust and water and building our highly complex cell parts, cells, and us out of our foods, it is easy to take His caring works for granted unless we pause to consider the cause.

How significant is it that no one else can make our grown foods and us out of dirt and water? Through seventy years of failed attempts to make a living cell out of elements, it is now verified that no humans have the superintelligence essential for these life-construction works. Evolution, by definition, has NO intelligence to use and is, therefore, factually falsified as both the origin and cause of Life.

Grown foods are always available at the grocery store (at least in our four focus nations) and He does not send any bills for any of His phenomenal atom assembly works of making us out of dust.

Another reason for not thinking of His huge care for us is that for over fifty years, our schoolteachers and professors in secular schools and colleges have been forced to teach us that "evolution" is the origin and cause of life and no Creator is needed or allowed.

This book provides simple, significant, scientific solutions to show why evolution is NOT the cause of life, but, as the majority of our citizens and governments have believed, God IS.

After decades of research and debate over God vs. Evolution as the cause of life, the massive accumulation of evidence regarding the complexity of living cell parts, cells, and entities, points to this verdict that is very simple: *evolution has no intelligence and without intelligence, you cannot build cell parts.* (See Chapter 3). The atoms for our body parts have to be found, carefully selected, counted, precisely assembled in sequence, and hooked up properly in order to function. Evolution cannot count, nor can it do any of the other superintelligent works with atoms that are essential for constructing and maintaining our cell parts, our cells, and us. By definition, evolution has no intelligence to use. Hopefully, scientists, teachers, and professors can soon stop having to pretend that no intelligence is needed and that, although living entities appear to be very obviously designed, *you must pretend they are not.* What a drastically misleading and confusing deception that has been forced on educators and students for over five decades.

Sources of Trouble from Within Our Western Society

The unscientific and misleading shortcomings of the evolutionary doctrine exclusively taught in our secular education institutions, were summed up by an open and honest evolutionist, Harvard's Professor Richard Lewontin. His words were, *"We take the side of* (evolutionary) *science in spite of the patent absurdity of some of its constructs, in spite of its failure to fulfill many of its extravagant promises of health and life, in spite of the tolerance of the scientific community for unsubstantiated just-so stories, because we have a prior commitment, a commitment to materialism. It is not that the methods and institutions of science somehow compel us to accept a material explanation of the phenomenal world, but, on the contrary, that we are forced by our a priori adherence to material causes to create an apparatus of investigation and a set of concepts that produce material explanations, no matter how counter-intuitive, no matter how mystifying to the uninitiated. Moreover, that materialism is absolute, for **we cannot allow a Divine Foot in the door."** *[1] (Emphasis added).

Disallowing students, teachers, and professors to follow the evidence wherever it leads is so obviously anti-science as well as anti-God of our nations. True science is to be encouraged to follow the evidence wherever it leads and to share the findings without reprisal.

Another major source of trouble is the "Humanist Project" that started in 1933. For example, atheists in the religion of Humanism expressed this message in their magazine, *The Humanist,* Jan.-

INTRODUCTION

Feb., 1983: *"The battle for mankind's future must be waged and won in the public-school classroom by teachers who correctly perceive their roles as the proselytizers of a new faith.... these teachers must embody the same selfless dedication as the most rabid fundamentalist preachers, for they will be ministers of another sort, utilizing the classroom instead of the pulpit to convey humanist values in whatever subject they teach, regardless of educational level - pre-school, day-care or large state university. **The classroom must and will become an arena of conflict** between the old and the new - the rotting corpse of Christianity, together with all its adjacent evils and misery, and the new faith of humanism."*

The humanists fail to mention the worldwide good works of unselfish Christians and Christian groups that feed the hungry, provide hospitals, medical treatments, save lives, provide shelters for the poor, and are the largest providers of charitable works worldwide. The teachings of Jesus are about peace, concern for others, salvation, and gratitude to our creator, food provider, maintainer and healer. Just beware of imposters who "talk the talk but do not walk the walk" of Jesus.

You can now rest assured that your ancestors were not some type of modified monkey as evolution postulates. There is no "common ancestor" but there is a common designer, builder, provider, and maintainer for all living entities, including us. (See "Exposing Subtle Satan's Powerful Ploy" p. 127).

It has been recently shown that the design and construction of all living entities requires intelligence at a level far above that of highly intelligent humans. This was 'proven,' unintentionally, but beyond a shadow of a doubt, by the three 2016 Nobel Prize Winners in Chemistry, as well as other chemists, including the James Tour Group at Rice University. Scientists of all stripes have been trying to produce a living cell from raw elements for seventy-plus years without success. We just do not have enough intelligence, e.g. we cannot come close to making a living food cell out of dirt.

INTRODUCTION

It is now known that superintelligence, far above that of mankind, is required to construct our cells, which are phenomenally complex even when compared to an entire city. To show some of the basic essential intelligence required to build a new cell, let's take a look at building a simple birdhouse in comparison: intelligent decisions, choices, and physical skills with suitable materials are essential for both.

The first decisions include what the builder wants the birdhouse or the new cell to be like when it is finished, i.e. the intelligent design. For our birdhouse or cell, the decision has to be made as to how large each one will be, what materials are required and available and from where they can be obtained, how many pieces of each material will be needed, where each piece will be placed, how each piece will be fastened in place, and for working cells, when and how the "breath-of-life" will be added to the inanimate building-block atoms. The building materials for each (boards for the birdhouse or atoms for the cell) have no life of their own. The birdhouse needs no internal machinery, but the cell certainly does. Each of the 40+ types of molecular machines required for our 200+ cell-types are highly complex, and each requires that special "breath-of-life" to be added to enable the cell to function.

For the birdhouse, the right materials, tools, fasteners, and finishes must be manufactured or located from a supplier, selected, delivered to the construction site, and the assembly skills must be available.

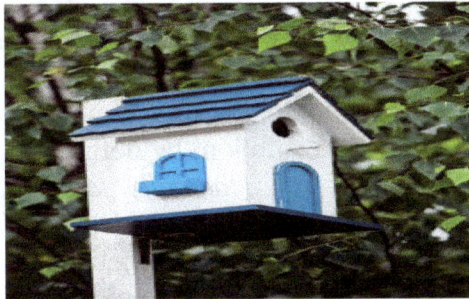

Alexander Tolstykh/Shutterstock

INTRODUCTION

For any one of our cells, the needed numbers of the correct types of atoms must be available from our digestive system, delivered and selected from the adjacent blood vessel, counted, then precisely assembled in sequence and fastened into the proper location in each cell part. These are all physical works with atoms that humans, as well as evolution, are incapable of performing.

ANATOMY OF A CELL

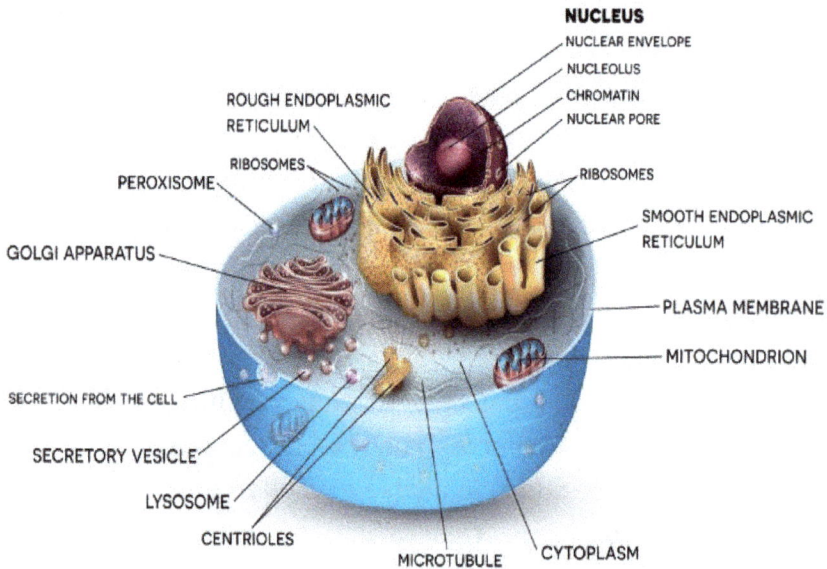

Tefi/Shutterstock

Building the birdhouse takes intelligence, but building the cell takes *superintelligence*. Humans have nowhere near enough intelligence nor construction skills to assemble atoms into all of the needed cell parts, and evolution, by definition, has no intelligence to use. Therefore, it is *factually falsified* as the cause required to design and build living cells with atoms from our foods. Other parts not shown include the DNA helix which is about two meters long with about six billion bases precisely arranged.

INTRODUCTION

In this book, you will find many fascinating details concerning *the phenomenal works and care our Creator provides for each one of us every second of every day.*

The study of these details has become the new life science for explaining how all Life is amazingly constructed and maintained by a brilliant being. This being is called "God" by our governments and the majority of our citizens.

This science is new to mankind, but our Creator has probably been using it since the beginning of His creation of living things.

The name given to this life science is "Atomic Biology," but don't let the name scare you because the basics are simple enough for a fifth-grader to understand, like this:

(1) all material things, including our cells, are made of atoms;

(2) superintelligence (far above mankind's level) is proven essential to find, sort, select, count, and precisely assemble in sequence, the correct numbers of the correct atoms to construct our cell parts, cells, and us;

(3) the essential "breath-of-life" must be added to each cell for it to live and function. When removed, the cell's life ends.

Those are the simple basics for creating living cells and entities. It is the brilliance of the designs and construction works for cells that is complex far above man's capability. Darwinian evolution, by definition having <u>no</u> intelligence to use, should now be assigned to the history department, *if Truth for Life is to be taught.*

The development of this life science began unintentionally in 1987 as a curiosity for a "new believer" by the name of Tom Rogers, living in North Vancouver, Canada.

From a background in engineering, manufacturing, research, and construction, one of his first questions was, "How does this 'Creator' actually build living entities, including us?"

Tom's awards in biology, chemistry, and physics gave him a foundation on which to build a new science as an independent science researcher. In addition, he has decades of experience with the practical work of designing and building things. An old adage regarding engineering's need to go far beyond theory is that "The bridge has to stand, and the plane has to fly!"

Tom has attended three universities plus two other institutes and states, "Although I do not have a PhD, I believe I have done the time (20 years part-time and 17 years full-time) and paid the price in costs and income forfeiture, for focusing, studying, researching, discovering, and developing this new God-based life science of Atomic Biology". Input has been gathered through and from a total of forty-five scholars in developing this life science.

Huge "thank you's" are especially due to co-authors Dr. Jerry Bergman and Dr. Graham McLennan as well as other directors, staff, and of course, wife Bonnie.

The BIG question is, "Since it can be shown that super-intelligent physical works are essential for building living cells and entities, does this falsify Darwinisms and all macro-evolutionary philosophies regarding the origin and cause of life?"

Many won't like the answer at first but it has become an obvious, *"Yes." We are all brilliantly created and cared for by our Creator.* Truth is always better to live by than falsehoods.

"God's Biology," the nickname for "Atomic Biology," is a culmination of over three decades of research including input from 20 PhDs, 9 DScs, 3 MDs, 3 Mathematicians, 2 MScs, and 8 Independent Researchers.

As with the Bible, some key concepts are repeated for emphasis. As a study/textbook, this book will probably be studied one chapter at a time.

Our driving belief is this: ***Citizens, including all our students, have the unalienable right to be taught Why God Is So Highly Recognized By Their Government, and what phenomenal scientific work and care He is providing for each one of us every second of every day.***

INTRODUCTION

This "Darwin's Replacement Series" is part of the "Truth For Life Education Project."

As the national governments of our focus nations (USA, UK, Australia, and Canada) all highly recognize our Creator, we often quote from His "operator's manual', the Holy Bible.

SCRIPTURES ON GOD'S
CREATIVE WORKS FOR US (from the NIV)

The following quoted scriptures are very clear from God's Word. The God we refer to is the triune God of our Western nations. He gives no mention of evolution or theistic evolution contributing in any way to the creation or reproduction of any living entities. He earns 100% of the credit for producing all grown foods out of dust and water and all Life from those foods. *Think of Him when you enter the grocery store and see the apples, oranges, potatoes and carrots, etc. that He has made for Your Life. Without His created foods, you would not exist.*

The following are God-inspired messages from His "operator's manual" for each of us for our best life. It contains history and great advice that our governments and citizens can benefit from immensely if we would just USE IT.

Genesis 1:21   So <u>God created</u> the great creatures of the sea, and every living and moving thing with which the water teems and that moves about in it, according to their kinds, and every winged bird according to its kind. And God saw that it was good.

Genesis 1:26   Then God said, "<u>Let us make mankind</u> in our image, in our likeness, and let them rule over the fish of the sea and the birds in the sky, over the livestock and all the wild animals, and over all the creatures that move along the ground."

INTRODUCTION

Genesis 1:27   So God created mankind in his own image, in the image of God he created them; male and female he created them.

Genesis 2:7   The Lord God formed the man from the dust of the ground and breathed into his nostrils the breath of life, and the man became a living being.

Genesis 2:22   Then the Lord God made a woman from the rib he had taken out of the man, and he brought her to the man.

Psalm 139: 13-14   For you created my inmost being; you knit me together in my mother's womb. I praise you because I am fearfully and wonderfully made; your works are wonderful, I know that full well.

Ecclesiastes 3:11   He has made everything beautiful in its time. He also set eternity in the hearts of men; yet they cannot fathom what God has done from beginning to end.

Isaiah 40:28   Do you not know? Have you not heard? The Lord is the everlasting God, the Creator of the ends of the earth. He will not grow tired or weary, and his understanding no one can fathom.

John 1:1-3   In the beginning was the Word, and the Word was with God, and the Word was God. He was with God in the beginning. Through him all things were made; without him nothing was made that has been made.

Romans 1:20   For since the creation of the world, God's invisible qualities -- his eternal power and divine nature---have been clearly seen, being understood from what has been made, so that people are without excuse.

Romans 11:36   For from him and through him and for him are all things. To him be the glory forever! Amen

Ephesians 2:10   For we are God's handiwork, created in Christ Jesus to do good works, which God prepared in advance for us to do.

SCRIPTURES ON SATAN'S
DESTRUCTIVE DEEDS

It seems that most of the members of our formerly great society have dropped their spiritual armor somewhere and thereby exposed themselves to Satan's deceptive and destructive tricks.

A recent Canadian study, "Hemorrhaging Faith," indicates that we the people, are largely to blame as we have allowed Satan to pull us away from God's guidance. According to the study, the four main mistakes we have allowed to go unchecked are those of hypocrisy, judgementalism, exclusivity, and failure to engage.

Going deeper to something that seems fearfully unmentionable is one of Satan's most powerful ploys: six decades of exclusive teaching in our public education systems that Darwinian evolution is the origin and cause of all life – no God is allowed!

How many souls have been dissuaded from believing that our Creator, the God of our nations (USA, UK, Canada, Australia, and more), is the True Creator, Sustainer, and Maintainer of all Life?

We can all take heart that *the Theories of Evolution are now factually falsified regarding both the origin and cause of Life. And this is the start of a very good reset for our society.* Only our superintelligent Creator has the ability essential to design and build all living cells for our grown foods and us.

He makes us out of dust and water, like this: From atoms in the dust, He makes living cells for all our grown foods and from those same atoms in our foods, He makes all our living cells and us.

However, *Satan really does not want people to know this.*

If anyone thinks that creating complex living cell parts, cells, and beings like us can just happen without any intelligence or enormous careful work, I suggest they honestly think this through. Watch for our coming book titled, *God Is In The Grocery Store.*

Let's look at some of God's words regarding subtle old Satan, Public Enemy #1, the Devil himself: (from the NIV).

Genesis. 3:1 Now the serpent (inhabited by Satan) was thus more crafty than any of the wild animals the Lord God had made. He said to the woman, "Did God really say, 'You must not eat from any tree in the garden?" (Inspiring doubt about God, like our public education system does today).

Zechariah 3:2 Then he showed me Joshua, the high priest, standing before the angel of the Lord, and Satan standing at his right side to accuse him.

Luke 22:3 Then Satan entered Judas, called Iscariot, one of the Twelve. (Inspiring betrayal of Jesus).

Acts 10:38 ...how God anointed Jesus of Nazareth with the Holy Spirit and power, and how He went around doing good and <u>healing all who were under the power of the devil</u> because God was with Him.

Romans 16:20 The God of peace will soon crush Satan under your feet.

2 Corinthians 11:3 But I am afraid that just as Eve was deceived by the serpent's cunning, your minds may somehow be led astray from your sincere and pure devotion to Christ.

2 Corinthians 11:14 And no wonder, for Satan himself masquerades as an angel of light.

Ephesians 4:27 ... and do not give the devil a foothold.

1 Timothy 1:20 Among them are Hymenaeus and Alexander, whom I have handed over to Satan to be taught not to blaspheme.

James 4:7 Submit yourselves, then, to God. Resist the devil, and he will flee from you.

1 Peter 5:8 Be alert and of sober mind. Your enemy, the devil, prowls around like a roaring lion looking for someone to devour.

If you are interested in helping to save our society from the destructive influences and forces of evil, please visit our website at www.atomicbiology.com and our "Truth For Life Education Project."

Remember: even Richard Dawkins, who has often spoken for the atheists of the world, has recently admitted that the loss of the influence of Christianity would be bad for society.[2] He now considers himself to be a "cultural Christian." [3]

Glossary

Normally, the glossary would be in the back of the book; however, some of our expanded definitions of old terms are new. Without having the definitions used by the authors, you would not receive clarity for the new information herein.

Although some of the terms may seem technical, you will find the book more enlightening and beneficial if you are familiar with the terms in this list. Many of these terms are interrelated.

Atomic Biology

This is the name that we, at Reality Research & Development, gave to the science of studying the enormous amount of superintelligent works essential for locating, sorting, selecting, counting, grasping, and precisely placing and fastening all of the right numbers of the right atoms in sequence as required for constructing, sustaining, growing, maintaining, and repairing living cells and living entities. This is a God-based life science.

With each discovery in science, it is becoming more apparent that most sciences are in fact, a study of God's essential, superintelligent inventions and careful works.

Do not be confused regarding the misused concept of separation of church and state. See "God" in this glossary.

Atoms

They are commonly referred to as the "building blocks of the universe." According to mainstream science, virtually all atoms are comprised of a nucleus made up of protons and neutrons with electrons being moved *perpetually* in orbits around the nucleus at a finely controlled speed so as not to fly out of orbit by being moved too quickly, nor to implode into the nucleus by being moved too slowly. Atoms have no *internal* means of self-directed movement; no legs, fins, wings, muscles, or brain, and therefore must rely on a profound *external force* to move them into their precise position in each living cell.

Biological Construction

This is the superintelligent physical work of building living cells and entities by finding, sorting, selecting, counting, grasping, and precisely assembling in sequence and fastening all the correct numbers of the correct atoms from available sources. These works are essential to building each complex part of every living cell, along with adding the necessary 'breath-of-life' to each cell, precisely programming its DNA and RNA to make it specifically functional, and assembling various specialized cells into the particular living entity desired by the builder.

Biomimicry

Is skillful work performed to duplicate useful things that are already designed and built by God and can be helpful for people.

"Breath-of-Life"

The incomparable basic necessity for life in every living cell, without which, no cell lives or functions.

Common Descent

The evolutionary concept stating that similarities between different kinds of plants and creatures indicate a "common ancestor."

However, a more scientific and logical understanding of the intelligent design, construction, sustenance, and maintenance work required for living entities reveals the necessity for a *brilliant common designer, builder, sustainer, and maintainer.*

Creation

The superintelligent work performed for the design, construction, sustenance, growth, maintenance, and repair of all living entities, by an omniscient being using elemental atoms.

Decisions and Choices for Cell Construction

Key factors in the work of assembling atoms into cell parts are the decisions for sequencing the assembly of the correct numbers of the right atoms, then choosing the right atoms from amongst the wrong ones and assembling them into each part of each cell with precise placement and bonding for each atom. It takes superintelligence to do this work and knowledge of how each part of each different cell has to function on completion. Think of the billions of intelligent decisions and choices necessary for finding, selecting, counting and assembling the right numbers of the right atoms for approximately six billion bases to build the DNA molecule in each cell. (See Chapter 3).

Design

The amazingly complex work of planning the layout and functions of each cell part and cell for each living entity, planning the source of the correct atoms for its building materials, planning the right numbers of the correct atoms to be selected from amongst millions of unsuitable atoms, planning the DNA programs for the functions of each cell part, plus engineering and building up to 40 of the various molecular machines essential for each different cell.

Energy

The perpetual power supplied consistently, carefully, and constantly to provide controlled perpetual motion to every electron in every atom. The amount of energy in a gram of matter could light up a city for weeks. The challenge is how to access all this energy. Atomic energy plants do quite a good job of this.

Evolution (Darwinian)

Because this topic is so crucial to understanding Life and so controversial, it is vitally important to any discussion of it that the individuals agree on which definition of 'evolution' they wish to discuss.

In this book, we are focused on the definition of Darwinian evolution that is compulsorily taught in our Western public education systems, from the upper biology curriculum establishers all the way down through the grades to where the origin and cause of life are first taught.

This definition includes a "universal common ancestor," which is an original cell that just happened to be assembled from non-living elements with no intelligence involved. This cell or entity would have needed to have the built-in capability to survive and reproduce offspring with improvements. These offspring would have needed reproductive ability to make other offspring with more improvements that would gradually lead to the reproduction of all living species of plants, bacteria, animals, birds, sea creatures, humans, and more.

Because of the extreme improbability for such a complex original life-form to "happen," many evolutionists, as well as former evolutionists, are realizing this concept for creating a life form is, in truth, impossible.

The theory that all of this "just happened" through Darwin's perception of "natural selection," **is now a factually falsified theory.** This is because it is now proven that we humans do not have anywhere near enough intelligence to build even the simplest living cell from atoms and Darwinian evolution, by definition, has **no** intelligence to use.

Because Darwinian evolution is taught exclusively, blocking the teaching of any intelligence-based life science, **it has become an anti-science.** It is an anti-science because it currently disallows basic true science which encourages the following of evidence wherever it leads and without reprisal.

God

The name given by English-speaking people and governments to the superintelligent and life-producing being who creates and sustains all living entities. He exists both in eternity and infinity in that there is no known beginning or end for Him. His intelligently controlled energy (see 'Perpetual Motion') is required to consistently move every electron in every atom in every element perpetually at the right speed. There is no other known source of this essential supply of controlled energy to cause this perpetual motion. This partially explains His omnipresence, and omniscience as He has a presence in all the atoms in all living cells. He alone has the essential superintelligence to be the brilliant designer, builder, sustainer, maintainer and repairer of every living cell in every living entity. This includes those cells in the food necessary for our life. He is the provider of the essential "breath of life" required by each cell of every living entity in order for it to live and function; no cell lives without it. He is the programmer of all DNA and RNA, and the builder of all the molecular machines and other complex parts for every cell. His phenomenal works, capabilities, and care seem unlimited except by His own will. This earns Him the description as omnipotent.

God is not to be confused with "the church" because a church can be a building or a group of people who are Satanists, Scientologists, Catholics, Protestants, Mormons, Jehovah's Witnesses, New Agers, cults, and even evolutionists who believe by faith, none of whom can create a single living thing.

"Separation of church and state" is not a law but a concept to prevent the state from dictating to churches what they are to do, and the church cannot dictate what the government is to do.

Remember that God is **not** the church, although He is a significant part of some churches, just as He is a significant part of most of our governments. His advice is worthy of our understanding, application, and benefit.

Students have the unalienable right to be taught why God is so highly recognized by their government, e.g. in Declarations, Pledges of Allegiance, Justice Systems, Nnational Holidays of Christmas, Easter, and Thanksgiving, in National ottos, on currencies, public buildings, war memorials, and more.

Intelligence

The ability to calculate the requirements for solutions to objectives and to provide the means to fulfill these requirements. Intelligence has to be far higher than mankind's level when it applies to the calculations, provisions, and works necessary to design and construct all living cell parts necessary for the life functions in every living entity. Scientists have proven over the last seventy-plus years that we do not have anywhere near enough intelligence to produce a living cell from elements. This is just one reason why we need our Creator God and His superintelligence.

Maintenance

In this book it means the intelligent work involved in sustaining, repairing, and maintaining cells for life in every living entity. This includes the delivery of the required form, type, and amount of energy necessary for each cell's requirements to function, the delivery of the correct type and amount of nourishment for its life, removing its waste products, and disposing of them through the entity's waste disposal system.

Molecular Machines

Of particular interest are the amazing tiny machines constructed within each of our cells to perform various critical functions.
The 2016 Nobel Prize for Chemistry was given to three scientists, J.P.Sauvage, Sir J.F.Stoddart, and B.L.Feringa, who had cooperatively researched and developed a few relatively simple molecular machines after over 30 years of research and development.

Even though these molecular machines required an enormous amount of scientific research, human intelligence, sophisticated equipment, and much time, they are extremely simple in comparison to any of the living molecular machines built for our cells, like kinesin, ribosomes, myosin, proteasomes, or splice-osomes, that God has to carefully construct for us within our new cells every day of the week.

Natural

An adjective to describe a temporary entity having limited lifespan and capability.

Natural Selection

A term used in Darwinism/macroevolution to describe the process that generates the survival-of-the-fittest organisms. It is a logical concept that those living entities with characteristics that weaken their capacity to survive (such as the inability to escape predators or obtain nutrients) will have less chance of reproducing and passing on their characteristics to succeeding generations.

Natural selection is also the theoretical "mechanism" for producing and maintaining life, however, it is not an intelligent force and does not have the required capabilities to do the essential intelligent work for constructing cells. These missing capabilities include: the intelligence to find, select, count, and assemble all the right numbers of the right atoms for cell part construction; the means of grasping atoms; the speed and dexterity for precisely placing the right numbers of the required atoms together to build all the cell parts; the intelligence to program DNA; and the power to provide the necessary "breath-of-life" without which *no cell can live or function*. In short, natural selection/evolution cannot construct, sustain, grow, maintain, and repair even one cell. In essence, it cannot perform any of these many superintelligent works necessary to create living entities. Many open-minded evolutionists and former evolutionists now acknowledge this fact.

There are thousands of scientists who are doubtful that evolution can create living entities, but the fear of penalty (job termination, loss of tenure or funding, besmirched reputation) by evolutionists in power, intimidates them from professing their doubts publicly.

This use of force and intimidation to prevent the following of scientific evidence to wherever it leads is clearly **anti-science** and should be outlawed.

Parameters of Possibility (for natural selection)

A limit to the capacity for accomplishment of objectives without superintelligent help. For example, if you have a large bowl full of marbles of ten different colors, how many groups of ten different colors do you think you could sort, select, pick out and place in a circular pattern in one second using your intelligence, eyesight, arms, and hands? Maybe two (if you are lucky)?

Now compare this to the work necessary just for the replacement of all our red blood cells about every 120 days. For just one average-sized human adult, *over forty-nine hundred quadrillion (4,900,000,000,000,000,000) correct atoms per second have to be sorted from his or her digesting food, then selected, counted, grasped, assembled into new red blood cells, and delivered into his or her bloodstream* (see Chapter 1 references).

Perpetual Motion

Electrons in atoms are constantly and consistently moved using the controlled energy supplied by the all-powerful being we call God. This energy applies to the movement of electrons virtually forever in all atoms. It is a phenomenal capability involving a carefully produced and controlled energy supply, intelligence, precision, consistence, and work. Perpetual motion is not possible without omniscient design and work.

Satan

A destructive spiritual being that tempts individuals to do things that cause trouble and later usually gives them deep regrets. He is the chief adversary of God and goodness. He is referred to as "Public Enemy #1" and probably played a role in having the Lord's Prayer and Bible reading of God's advice removed from public education in the mid-1960s.

It is difficult to imagine how much trouble and heartache this has caused members of our society over the years.

In fact, it is possible that Satan's most damaging ploy has been his influence on education to substitute God's enormous work and care for every person, with Darwin's Godless Theory of Evolution for the origin and cause of Life.

A lot more focus on Satan's temptations into trouble should be taught in our classrooms.

Selection

The deliberate and intelligent choosing of the right numbers of the right atoms as part of the work essential to build, sustain, grow, maintain, and repair living entities. This work cannot be performed except by a superintelligent entity.

Superintelligent

An adjective that describes the perpetual being that has abilities which immensely surpass human intelligence, dexterity, capability, speed, and endurance. See the definition of *God.*

Superintelligent Reliability

A characteristic of the consistently predictable, hyper-intelligent works provided by the Designer, Builder, Sustainer, and Maintainer of all living entities. A few examples we can rely on Him for are:

- *gravity* to keep material items like us from flying off the face of the Earth as it spins on its axis;

- *sunlight* for warmth, energy, and its part in the growth and maintenance of living entities;
- the *repositioning and healing effect of pharmaceutical atoms* ingested to help healing and to relieve pain;
- the *building* of Red Delicious apples when Red Delicious apple seeds are planted, tomatoes when tomato seeds are planted, carrots when carrot seeds are planted, and so on.

All of these *and much more* are critical to Life, yet because of God's amazing reliability and consistency, all these brilliant works and care for us are too often taken for granted.

Sustenance

The foods and beverages created by God for the nourishment of each and every one of His plants and creatures. From the available sources of the right numbers of the right atoms. He sorts, selects, grasps, and precisely assembles right atoms to make these foods and beverages for use by His creatures especially in developing energy for warmth and mobility of all muscles, for growth, for maintaining and repairing cells, for the phenomenal abilities to think, live, function, etc.

Works

The superintelligent efforts of a supreme mind are essential in the careful work of designing, building, growing, sustaining, maintaining, and repairing each living entity as the Builder chooses.

References and Notes:

[1] Lewontin, R., *Billions and Billions of Demons*, The New York Review of Books, New York, NY, 9 January, 1997.

[2] https://www.breitbart.com/national-security/2016/01/12/professional-atheist-dawkins-says-christianity-bulwark-against-something-worse/

[3] Hobson, T., *Is Richard Dawkins a Christian?* spectator.co.uk, 2 April, 2024.

Part I:

Introducing the new Life science of "Atomic Biology" (nicknamed "God's Biology").

Its goal is to replace Darwinisms as the taught origin and cause of Life and in Truth, to bring 100% of the credit for producing all Life back to our Creator, the God of our nations.

INTRODUCTION

Chapter 1

The Essentiality of a Super-Intelligent Creator for Our Life

Quotes from Charles Darwin:

"...the Works of the Creator are (superior) to those of man." [1]
(He did have this part of his story of life right for a time).

"But just in proportion as this process of extermination has acted on an enormous scale, so must the numbers of intermediate varieties, which have formerly existed, be truly enormous. Why then is every geological formation and every stratum not full of such intermediate links? Geology assuredly does not reveal any such finely graduated organic chain; and this perhaps is the most obvious and serious objection which can be urged against my theory [of evolution]." [2]

"To suppose that the eye with all its inimitable contrivances for adjusting the focus to different distances, for admitting different amounts of light, and for the correction of spherical and chromatic aberration, could have been formed by natural selection, seems, I freely confess, absurd in the highest degree" [3]

"If it could be demonstrated that any complex organ could not possibly have been formed by numerous successive slight modifications, my theory would absolutely break down." [4]

Quotes from scientist I. L. Cohen:

"At that moment, when the RNA/DNA system became under-stood, the debate between Evolutionists and Creationists should have come to a screeching halt." [5]

(He rightfully shows that when the enormous and superintelligent complexities of RNA and DNA programming were discovered, the theory of evolution, which, by definition, has no intelligence to program with, should have been immediately discarded).

"Any suppression which undermines and destroys that very foundation on which scientific methodology and research were erected, evolutionist or otherwise, cannot and must not be allowed to flourish. ...It is a confrontation between scientific objectivity and ingrained prejudice – between logic and emotion – between fact and fiction. ...In the final analysis, objective scientific analysis has to prevail – no matter what the final result is – no matter how many time-honored idols have to be discarded in the process.... It is not the duty of science to defend the theory of evolution, and stick by it to the bitter end – no matter what illogical and unsupported conclusions it offers... If in the process of impartial scientific logic, they find that creation by outside superintelligence is the solution to our quandary, then let's cut the umbilical cord that tied us down to Darwin for such a long time. It is choking us and holding us back.

*...Every single concept advanced by the theory of evolution (and amended thereafter) is imaginary as it is not supported by the scientifically established facts of microbiology, fossils, and mathematical probability concepts. Darwin was wrong. **The theory of evolution may be the worst mistake (ever) made in science.**"* [6] (Emphasis added).

The Theory of Evolution (i.e., 'macroevolution') is based on the wrong premise that since minor changes in a species can occur from generation to generation (i.e.,'microevolution'), then major changes can accumulate over a long period of time, changing one kind of creature into another kind. Some believe this could lead to entirely new species that are the result of the fittest survivors being selected naturally while the less fit do not survive.

On the surface, this seems logical and straightforward. Theoretically, no intelligent creation is required. Entities reproduce naturally, and all living species ascended from a tiny "common ancestor" according to Darwin's "Tree of Life."

However, *this theory conveniently overlooks several major essentials,* some of which are now recognized even by evolutionists and former evolutionists, for example, the now-understood phenomenal complexity that would have been required by the original "common ancestor" and the awesome complexity essential in the construction of all cell parts and cells.

We will show that even micro-evolution (intra-species variation) does not 'just happen' without the superintelligent physical work required for finding, sorting, selecting, counting, and precisely placing in sequence all the right numbers of the needed various elemental atoms from available sources. This work is essential to construct every complex part of every cell. Then, the "breath of life" has to be added to these inanimate atoms to make the cell parts function. When this is removed, the cell's life is over.

Our 200+ different types of cells also require up to 40 highly complex and guided molecular machines to be constructed within them. The James Tour Group knows how much intelligence it takes to design and build even the simplest molecular machines. You can also read about the intelligent physical work it took for Jean-Pierre Sauvage, Sir John Fraser Stoddart, and Bernard L. Feringa to build simple molecular machines before winning the 2016 Nobel Prize in Chemistry.

In spite of the 33 years of costly and complicated work needed to develop these tiny units, they are absolutely simplistic compared to any of the molecular machines constructed for our new cells, including kinesin, ribosomes, myosin, proteasomes, spliceosomes, cohesin, and about 35 others. (See Chapter 5).

Evolution cannot even begin doing this superintelligent cell construction work, as, by definition, it has no intelligence to use.

THE ESSENTIALITY OF A SUPER-INTELLIGENT CREATOR FOR OUR LIFE

Having no intelligence, "evolution" cannot even count, and if you cannot count atoms, you cannot build cell parts.

The God-based life science of "Atomic Biology" we are introducing includes Intelligent Design but goes far beyond design through the enormous amount of essential superintelligent physical works with atoms that must be performed in constructing, sustaining, maintaining, repairing, and replacing the cell parts and cells of creatures including us.

Atomic Biology goes beyond information to decisions, choices, and precision works. It goes far beyond the parameters of possibility for natural selection and random mutation to reveal the true cause of life.

It is our goal to combine all these concepts into one science that details the amazing caring work of creating, sustaining, and maintaining each living entity. Logically, "Atomic Biology" will be that life science.

Our focus at The Atomic Biology Institute is not on the unknown dates when life began on Planet Earth, but on understanding the details necessary for living cells and entities to be assembled, sustained, maintained, repaired, and replaced, *today.* A prime example of God's type of observable macro-evolution is the changing of a relatively unattractive *crawling* creature into a beautiful *flying* butterfly within 12 to 14 days, not millions of years.

Such is His amazing work in dissembling a *crawling* caterpillar down to an atomic soup in a chrysalis, then brilliantly reassembling most of the same atoms into a beautiful *flying* butterfly. We have a name for this work, "metamorphosis," but the name does not do the essential demolition and reconstruction work; our Creator does.

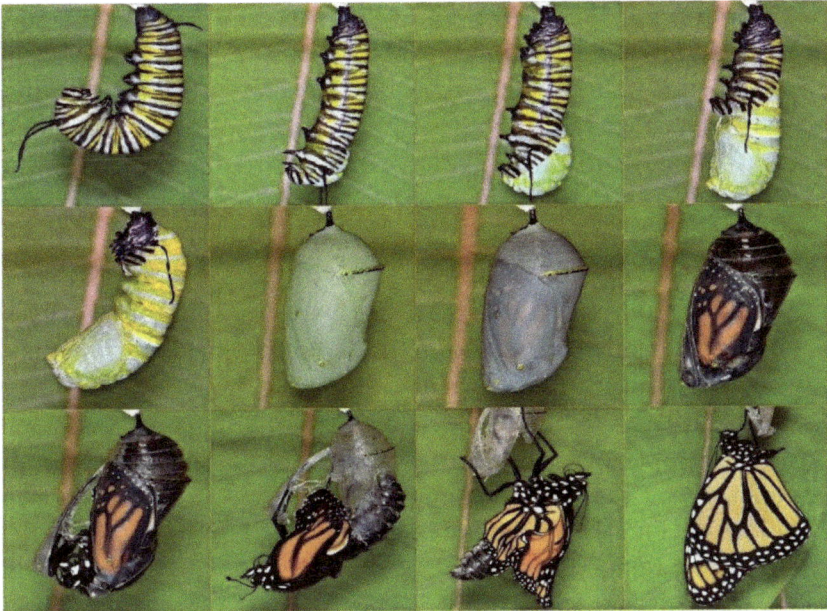

Stephen Russell Smith Photos/Shutterstock.com

Building humans from "the dust" is a far more awesome and complex task. The concept is simple, but the work is virtually miraculous.

If you look at any group of cells in your body, e.g. skin cells, eye cells, foot cells, nose cells, you can ask, "From where did the atoms come for these cells?"

Answer: From the food we consumed and a little from the air we breathed.

"And from where did those food atoms come?"

Answer: From the soil and moisture in gardens, fields, and orchards, and a little from the air.

This is why we know we are made from dust, like this: atoms in the soil are used to make our food, and then many of the same atoms in our food are assembled into our cells and us.

But "How" God does this work is the phenomenally complex part. It takes far more intelligence, dexterity, design, decisions, choices, speed, and precise sequential construction work, than scientists can come anywhere near. This is one of the reasons why Darwin was right when he said in *Origins*, "... *the works of the Creator are (superior) to those of man.*"[1] even though he did not know all the details. (We believe he was later 'persuaded' to ignore this viewpoint for many years).

We will provide more of the basic details of life within this book. The more we learn about the marvelous molecular machines built into our cells to do the variety of works required therein, the more the case is strengthened, not for a common ancestor, but for a common designer, builder, and maintainer of all living entities.

This book will help to clarify some of the great benefits in understanding our Creator's immense care for each one of us. As mentioned in the Introduction, the God of our Governments in these four nations, is the triune God of the Bible. He is not to be confused with "the church," as a church can be a building or a group of people who are Satanists, Scientologists, New Agers, Catholics, Protestants, Mormons, Jehovah's Witnesses, cults, evolutionists, etc. No church can create any living entity. God is definitely *not* "the Church."

God is, however, a significant part of some churches, just as He is a significant part of our governments as shown by His inclusion in national holidays (Christmas, Good Friday, Easter Monday, Thanksgiving, Christmas), in anthems ("God Save The King", "God Bless America, "God Keep Our Land Glorious and Free"), in declarations, pledges of allegiance, constitutions, oaths of office, on currencies ("In God We Trust," "Dei Gratia Regina"), on public buildings, war memorials, in national prayers, to name a few.

We must never lose our beneficial respect, acknowledgment, and appreciation for our Creator, Provider, and best Advisor. The central theme for the basic science chapters is to show a portion of the enormous amount of amazing and caring physical work involved in designing, constructing, and maintaining each unique one of us. We want to show the phenomenal design, intelligence, speed, dexterity, and reliable work and care required to find, sort, select, count, grasp, and precisely assemble the huge numbers of the required atoms to build each highly complex part of each of our individual cells. There are approximately 100 trillion functioning cells magnificently made and placed precisely in our body. They are amazingly connected to our blood system for nourishment, waste removal, repairs, replacement, and temperature control for each one of us. Also, our cells are carefully hooked up to our created thousands of miles of nerve systems, and electrical systems for muscle actions, problem monitoring, and internal communication for all our senses and reactions. Our cells are wonderfully and carefully assembled to create each one of us as a uniquely special human being.

Similar superintelligent physical work is performed for all creatures and plants, and we humans are given dominion over them all. May we gain the wisdom needed to do this well.

We must remember that atoms, of which every material thing is made, do not have legs, muscles, or brains. They cannot jump into their precise position in any cell because they do not have the internal means to do this. Of necessity, they require an *external entity* with capabilities that go far, far, far beyond any unguided process like Darwinian evolution.

This external being must construct our required foods using elements in the soil, air, and moisture in our fields, gardens, and orchards. Once we have consumed our food, this entity must arrange digestion and delivery of the atoms by our blood stream to each cell site for the construction of each highly complex part of the cell. Then each newly created cell requires the "breath of life" to be added because atoms have no life of their own. Of course, this phenomenal source is our creator whom we and our governments call "God." He is always within us caring for us.

This chapter could contain many volumes of detailed lists yet still miss huge numbers of the amazing works our Creator and Sustainer performs for us every second of every day.

Let's consider some of His phenomenal *work and care* for us humans plus other marvelous creatures and plants He has made.

1. He Builds Our Best Foods

This essential work is performed for us on a daily basis. As soon as we recognize that material things including our foods are made of atoms and that atoms do not have legs or any other <u>internal means</u> to move themselves from their position in the soil, air, or moisture to their precise position in each cell for each morsel of our grown food, we can understand why *a superintelligent <u>external entity</u>* is necessary.

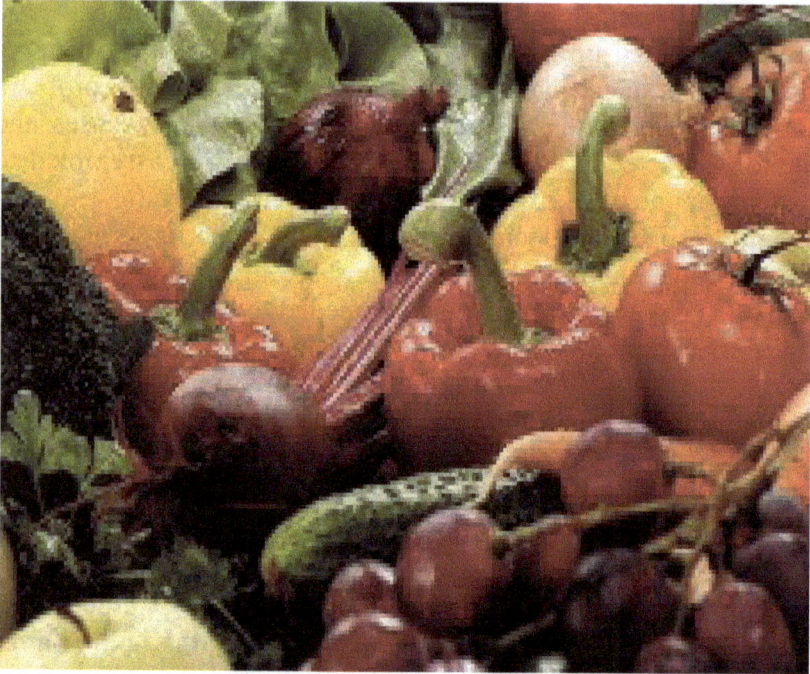

monticello/shutterstock.com

This applies not only to each cell of every tiny root, and to the body of each vegetable or fruit, but to the leaves as well. There are multi-millions of various cells in each morsel of food, and each cell requires billions of the right atoms to be precisely placed and fastened.

Cell construction, including the programming of DNA in each cell, does not happen by magic, magnetism, chemical reactions, electronics, or evolution. It requires a huge amount of super-intelligent, physical work and care at each cell-construction site.

The amount of food manufactured from the soil, air, and water around the world has to be sufficient to feed, without stopping, each one of us and our more than eight billion global neighbors, every day of every year. Think about this vast work and care for a moment.

This is the main reason why our national governments established a special holiday to give thanks to our Creator and Sustainer for all His caring work for us. It is called "Thanks-giving Day".

Some of us give thanks to this wonderful Provider, at every mealtime.   We *could* learn to share our foods much better.

2. He Builds Our Babies and Our Bodies

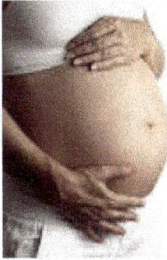

shutterstock · 81377626

Aaron Amat

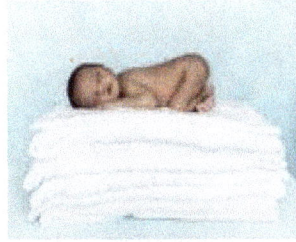

shutterstock · 140065822

Anneka

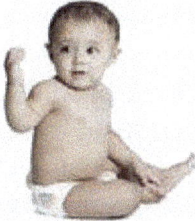

shutterstock · 163052954

imaged.com

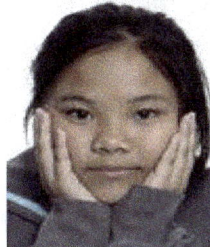

shutterstock · 54981316

naluwan

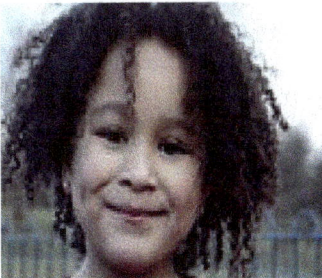

shutterstock · 47072353

kenny 1

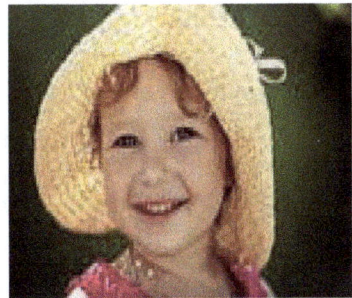

shutterstock · 150360296

lemuana

THE ESSENTIALITY OF A SUPER-INTELLIGENT CREATOR FOR OUR LIFE

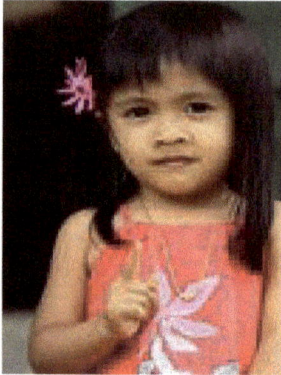

Studio One/ Shutterstock.com

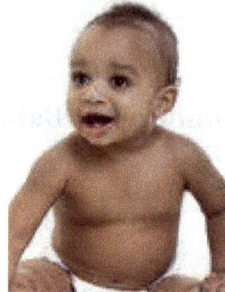

Samuel Borges
Photography

Who among us does not marvel at the birth of a baby? We recognize this as a wondrous event. Why should we have to pretend they are not designed, as the atheistic teachers insist?

A seven-pound (3.2 kg) newborn baby has been constructed over a nine-month period from two combined seeds, an egg and a sperm, plus quadrillions of the right atoms selected from the food the mother has consumed. It stands to reason that each of the correct atoms has been found, counted, grasped, precisely placed, and fastened to build each complex cell complete with its molecular machinery in operation. A baby is made with trillions of newly constructed cells. Just **one** red blood cell, for example, is made of approximately 280,000,000 molecules of hemoglobin x 10,000 atoms per molecule = 2,800,000,000,000 (twenty-eight hundred billion) of the correct atoms per red blood cell.

The wrong numbers and/or the wrong atoms would not work. We in science do not have enough intelligence to build even one living molecular machine for any cell, so why would we think that a theoretical process with **no** intelligence could? Even the best scientists in the field cannot build a single living cell out of elements, like building a carrot root cell out of dirt and water.

The volume, speed, precision, dexterity, and brilliance required to do this work is so awesome, essential and reliable that it really should be personally appreciated, if not revered.

Since it happens so consistently and reliably, we can easily take it for granted. However, this requires an enormous amount of caring and highly complex, physical work that evolution is not capable of performing as it possesses no care or intelligence.

3. He Builds Our Astounding Brains

According to Professor Paul Reber of Northwestern University the human brain consists of about one billion neurons, each of which forms about 1000 connections and each neuron can connect with other neurons. As he stated in the June 2010 issue of *Scientific American,* this results in "…exponentially increasing the brain's memory storage capacity to something closer to around 2.5 petabytes (or a million gigabytes)." [7] Reber compares this to about three million hours of recorded TV shows. With this much storage, the recorder could play continuously for over 300 years.

Van Wedeen and L.L. Wald of the Martinos Center for Biomedical Imaging Human Connectome Project state that "The brain's many regions are connected by some *100,000 miles* of fibres called white matter, enough to circle the Earth four times" [8]

Jeff Lichtman, a Harvard neuroscientist, is studying brain compositions. He was interviewed by Carl Zimmer who then wrote in *National Geographic*, February 2014, "So far the largest volume of a mouse's brain that Lichtman and his colleagues have managed to re-create is about the size of a grain of salt. Its data alone total a hundred terabytes, the amount of data in about 25,000 high-definition movies." They also indicate in the article that a mouse's brain contains about 70,000,000 neuron connections and a human brain contains about 1000 times that number. [9]

Douglas Axe, PhD, is an engineer-turned-molecular-biologist and former director of the Biologic Institute. In his recent book, *"Undeniable: How Biology Confirms Our Intuition That Life Is Designed,"* he reminds us that, *"The human brain is different…. Being the most remarkable component of the human body, it is arguably the most outstanding physical invention ever to exist."* [10]

This phenomenal computer, our brain, also had to be supremely built of atoms from the soil, air, and water with God's phenomenal two-step process: (1) Atoms in the soil built into food, then (2) those same atoms in our food are used to build our brain cells.

Where else would these atoms come from, and who else has the superintelligence to assemble them in such a phenomenal manner?

4. He Builds Our Pets

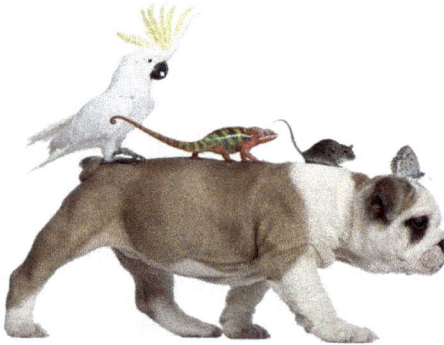

Susan Smitz/Shutterstock.com

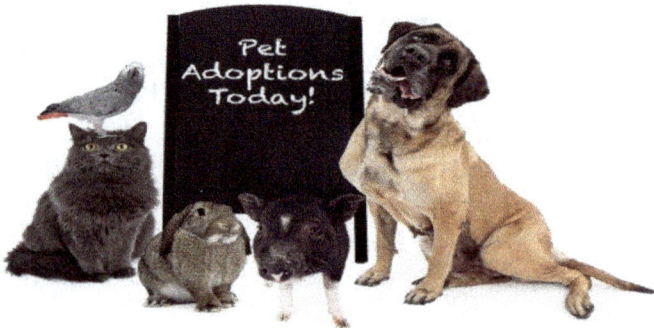

Eric Isselee/Shutterstock.com

Using exactly the same mind-boggling, planning, vision, technology, precision, dexterity, and care, God builds all other creatures as He builds us. None of us can come anywhere close to doing this brilliant work.

5. He Builds Beautiful Flowers For Our Enjoyment

Have you ever marveled at the beautiful colors, amazing fragrance, and functional design of some glorious flowers, and wondered how they could be made out of dirt? Does this not seem miraculous?

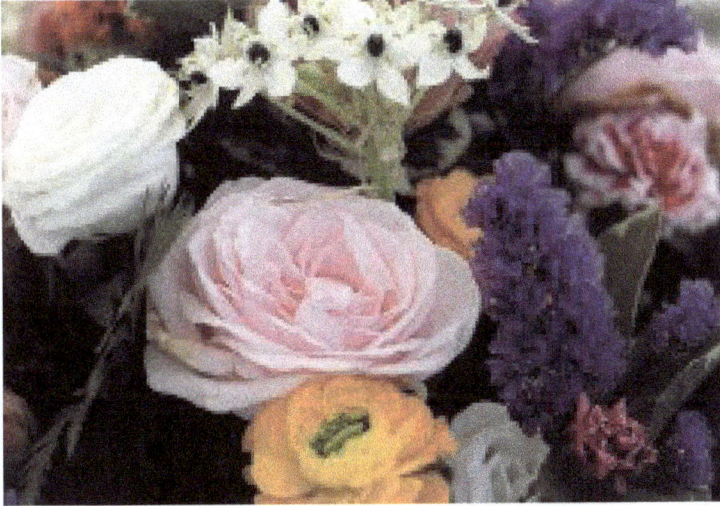

Flik47/shutterstock.com

6. He Builds Beautiful Fish

As God builds land creatures from the available atoms on land, so does He build beautiful sea creatures from atoms in the sea and in lakes and streams.

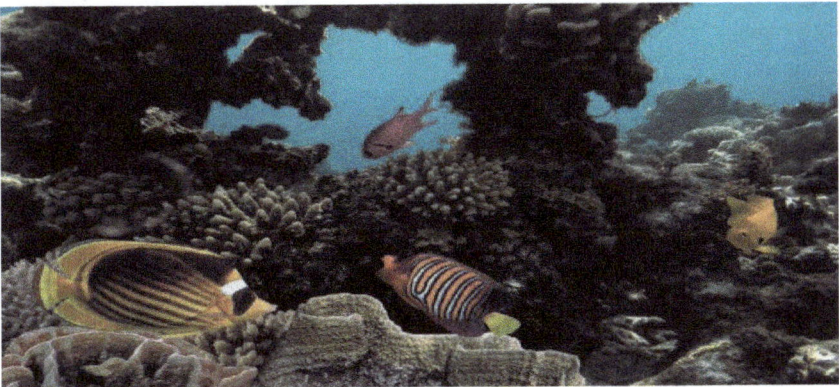

Vlad61/shutterstock.com

7. He Builds Beautiful Birds for Our Enjoyment

Do we marvel at the amazing colors of different birds, at some of their intriguing songs and calls, and at their wonderful ability to fly?

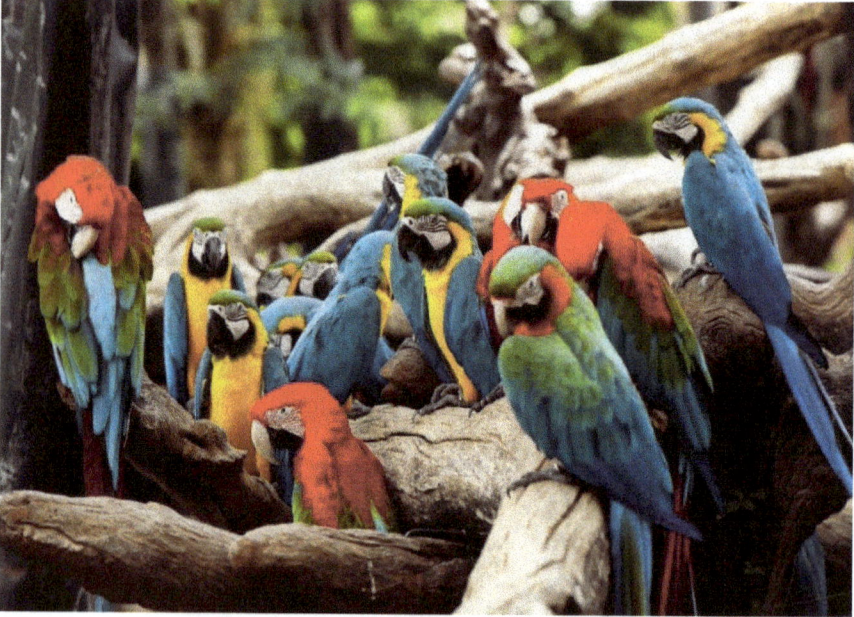

nattanan726/shutterstock.com

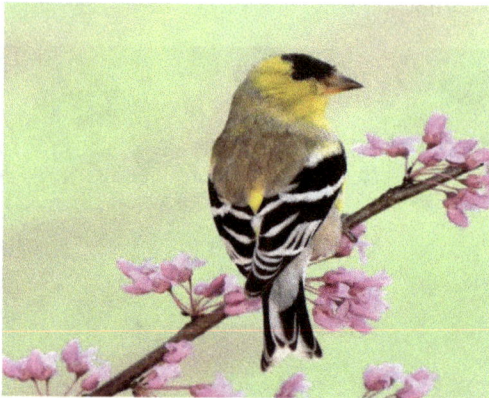

Stephen Russell Smith Photos/Shutterstock.com

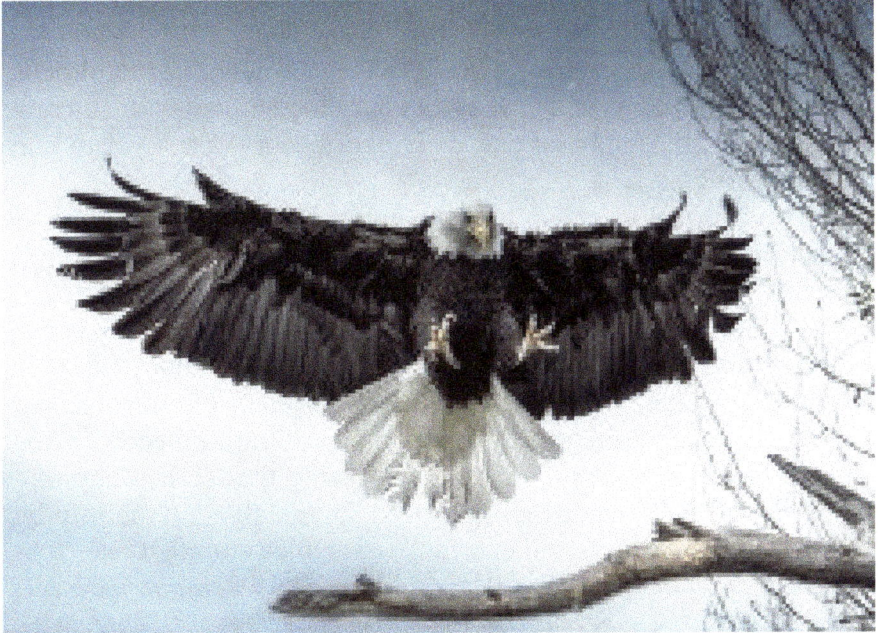

Phillip Rubino/Shutterstock.com

8. He Works So Caringly for Us

Building each one of us plus our foods, pets, flowers, and all life, is no simple task *(the understatement of life)*.

Since the concept of "atomic biology" is relatively new, many of the exact details regarding the right numbers and types of the elemental atoms required to build each type of our various cell parts are yet to be discovered. However, the cell composition we *have* analyzed can give us clues as to the work required in other cells.

In 2007 we calculated, with the help of C.J. Pallister, G.J. Tortora, and Max Perutz,[11] that to manufacture the enormous number of replacement red blood cells for an average person, over 4,900 quadrillion (4,900,000,000,000,000,000) *of the right elemental atoms* have to be found *every second* in our blood system which were picked up from our digestive system, delivered to our blood cell construction sites, then sorted, selected, counted, grasped, precisely placed, and fastened, with the special breath-of-life added.

Every second, each of these 2,000,000+ new red blood cells has to be completed and moved into our bloodstream with as many old ones being removed and delivered to our waste system and other areas.

This may be less than half the number of atoms that must be precisely placed for building our replacement red blood cells because, in the same second, a greater number of atoms (4900 quadrillion+ for fruit or vegetables including unused leaves, roots, etc.) have to be found in the soil in various gardens and fields, then sorted, selected, counted, grasped, then precisely placed and fastened to manufacture the food for each future second's red blood cells for each of us. This may bring the total to approx.-imately 10,000 quadrillion required atoms that are faithfully, precisely, constantly, and carefully assembled for each one of us *every second of every day, just to replace our worn-out red blood cells.*

How can anyone believe that this enormous and superintelligent physical work can be performed so reliably using no intelligence or care whatsoever?

In addition, at least 80 trillion (80,000,000,000,000) other cells in each adult are constantly and carefully sustained, maintained, repaired, or replaced.

There are so many other cell types to build and sustain for each of us: for eyelashes, hair, skin cells of various colors, to heart, lung, liver, and brain cells, to name a few of our 200+ different types of cells.

God also makes herbs and other special plant items that have been used for healing for centuries.

Many of our pharmaceuticals come from plants. There are even plant remedies which cure some types of cancer as noted by Suzanne M. Diamond, MSc, see *Canada's Amazing Anti-Cancer Tea!* [12] Another great article by Diamond outlining the special remedial effects of some of God's custom-built foods for us is "Humble Herbs Worth Their Weight in Gold", published in a 2008 issue of *Total Health Magazine.* [13]

She has also written an informative book, *Nature's Best Heart Medicine,* that outlines new scientific discoveries revealing how flavonoids are beneficial for people with heart disease, high blood pressure, varicose veins, circulation problems, and more.[14] We believe that determining the exact numbers and types of elemental atoms in each type of cell will be a great benefit in the development of more nutritional foods, and new pharmaceuticals to supply for use in the repair of cells that need to be healed. The information will also help in developing improved fertilizers that will contain all the necessary elements for optimal growth of our foods. There could be other attributes to the discovery of this information that would be beneficial for our health and healing. The logic is simple and understandable when you consider the following aspects of Atomic Biology:

Every material thing, including each of our cell parts, is made of atoms. If we determine exactly how many atoms of each type of element are in each kind of our healthy cells, and we determine if any one of our cells is experiencing problems because it lacks a portion of some elemental atoms, we could make sure there are enough of those types of atoms available to be placed into those cells for healing;

When we determine which foods contain an abundance of the atoms our unhealthy cells require, we can be sure to eat enough of them.

Conversely, if we have a tumor or other unwanted growth, we may determine the elements in that growth and find a way to prevent those elements from reaching the site. One view is that cancer requires high levels of glucose, so reducing glucose in the diet and cancer area, may help to shrink the cancer growth.

When we determine what atoms make up each healthy fruit, vegetable, nut, etc., we can make sure that there is an abundant supply of those atoms in the soil where the atoms have to be selected to build the specific food item. Suitable fertilizer could be added if the soil is analyzed and found to be lacking enough of the right necessary atoms for the food items to be optimally built, such as selenium, chromium, iron, or other common examples. Using the correct soil enhancers for building healthy food cells is like using good foods to supply enough of the required atoms for our Creator to build healthy cells for our us.

This enormous, brilliant, reliable, careful, and trustworthy work of building our foods and our cells is performed for each of us free of charge every second of our whole lifetime.

These are just a few of the logical reasons for Thanksgiving, and being grateful makes us happier. In spite of our relatively small problems, we all have so many blessings to be grateful for.

Many of us "give thanks" and say prayers at every meal. In addition, even though we do not share our resources very well, God *does* manufacture enough food for all eight+ billion of us every day.

Consider the enormous amount of work necessary to find, sort, select, count, and precisely assemble in sequence all the right numbers of the correct atoms of about 60 different elements from the soil that we need from our foods. Then, consider all the similar work needed to make all our 100 trillion cells from our foods. This could boggle one's mind but "Praise the Lord" for his massive and faithful works for us.

All of these atoms had to be created. They contain electrons that must be moved around the nucleus at precisely the right speed virtually forever. This perpetual motion is not a natural phenomenon; perpetual, ultra-intelligent control of the energy needed is also His work.

Then, for us to exist, we need the following:
1. The right amount of sunlight to grow our foods and help us to see the outside world, and to help keep us warm enough but not too warm, and just enough lunar gravity to help raise and lower the tides to refresh our oceans;
2. Enough good air to breathe with enough oxygen atoms and other air-born atoms necessary for our life;
3. A system to take the carbon dioxide we exhale and convert it into oxygen for us to inhale is exactly what our Creator designed plants and trees to do for us;
4. In addition, all the other essential details for life must be kept in balance and finely tuned (see Chapter 7).

It is easy to see that the vast amount of caring work for us humans is absolutely awesome. He does all this amazing work continuously for each one of us, whether we thank Him or not.

Does God *Deserve* Our Appreciation?

Might He be aggravated if He does not receive at least some "Thanksgiving" from each of us? (See Isaiah 42:8 and 48:11 to answer these questions).

How might He feel when the credit for all His enormous and caring works for us is given to something else like an idol or evolution? He says in many places in His Word, the Bible, that this eventually makes Him angry, and His anger has consequences. Is that understandable? Is that what Hell is for?

Applications for Life:

1. Which two groups of scientists are described for proving mankind does not have enough intelligence or ability to build the complex molecular machines for our cells?

_____

_____

2. How long does it take our Creator to "evolve" a *crawling* worm into a *flying* butterfly? _____

3. Does learning about the essential superintelligent work and care provided for you every second of every day, give you a sense of gratitude? Why? _____

_____

4. Does the theory that *no intelligence is required* for building beautiful birds, fish, flowers, and us, using atoms, seem logical to you? Why?_____

_____

5. What key factor did I.L. Cohen use to refute evolution as the cause of life? _____

_____

6. Explain why God and "the church" are not the same?

_____

_____

7. Who were the three Nobel Prize winners who worked 33 years to make molecular machines? How close did they come to making the complex molecular machines that our Creator makes for us every day?

_____

_____

_____

References and Notes:

[1] Darwin, Charles, *On the Origin of Species by Means of Natural Selection,* 1st edition, John Murray, London, England, 1859, p. 189: available online from Darwin-online.org.uk.

[2] Ibid., p. 280.

[3] Ibid., p. 186.

[4] Ibid., p. 189.

[5] Cohen, I.L., *Darwin was Wrong—A Study in Probabilities,* New Research Publications, New York, NY, 1984, p.5.

[6] Ibid., pp. 209–210.

[7] Reber, Paul, "What Is the Memory Capacity of the Human Brain," *Scientific American,* May/June 2010, www.scientificamerican.com/article/what-is-the-memorycapacity/.

[8] Wedeen, Van and L.L.Wald in article "Secrets of the Brain" by Carl Zimmer, *National Geographic,* February 2014, p. 34.

[9] Lichtman, Jeff in article "Secrets of the Brain" by Carl Zimmer in *National Geographic,* February 2014, pp. 39, 43.

[10] Axe, Douglas, *Undeniable,* Harper One, New York, NY, 2016, p.259

[11] Pallister, C.J., *Haematology: Biomedical Science Explained,* Butterworth-Heinemann, Burlington, MA, 1999. He states that an average 70 kg adult male produces *(or has produced for him)* about 2,300,000 red blood cells every second. Tortora, G. J., *Principles of Anatomy and Physiology,* John Wiley & Sons, New York, NY, 2008. He states that there are approximately 280,000,000 molecules of hemoglobin per red blood cell.

Perutz, Max, *Science is Not a Quiet Life: Unraveling the Atomic Mechanism of Hemoglobin,* World Scientific, Hackensack, NJ, 1997. He states that each hemoglobin molecule contains approximately 10,000 atoms.

If you do the math, you will find that the number of atoms required to be sorted from our eaten food, then selected, counted, grasped, and assembled into new red blood cells and delivered into our bloodstream is approximately $2,300,000 \times 280,000,000 \times 10,000 = 6,440,000,000,000,000,000$ (6,440 quadrillion) atoms every second of every day.

That approximate number is required for each average body every second of every day just for replacement red blood cells (based on a 70 kg. [154 lb.] male as average). We have conservatively used the figure of "over 4,900 quadrillion atoms per second" to include each of virtually all adults in the world.

[12] Diamond, Suzanne M., "Canada's Amazing Anti-Cancer Tea," *Common Ground,* December 1999, pp. 18,19.

[13] Diamond, Suzanne M., "Humble Herbs Worth Their Weight in Gold," *Total Health Magazine,* July/August 2008 issue.

[14] Diamond, Suzanne M., *Nature's Best Heart Medicine,* The Book Publishing Company, Summertown, TN, 2008.
https://bookpubco.com/products/natures-best-heart-medicine.

THE ESSENTIALITY OF A SUPER-INTELLIGENT CREATOR FOR OUR LIFE

Chapter 2:

What Happens at Our Cell Construction Sites?

Let's mentally become nano-observers and journey into the flesh near the end of a seven-year-old boy's forefinger. We will call him 'Johnny' and, of course, he is still growing.

We could pick an adult for our example because we receive new cells regularly. Nonetheless, Johnny's growing body provides us with a better observation site.

What we are looking at is a new cell construction site near the end of his finger. (You can look at your own forefinger and imagine the same work going on there.) We can watch the Builder's work in progress as He goes about His brilliant, rapid, and careful work involving decisions and choices plus selection and precise assembly in the proper sequence of the correct numbers of the required atoms and molecules for each new cell part.

Although most cells appear just to divide, an enormous number of physical works with atoms are involved. Before cell 'division' is finished, a new complete cell must be constructed connecting to the original cell which has to be left as a completed cell itself. Two different types of "cell divisions" exist, one called "mitosis" in which God uses parts of one cell to begin constructing a second cell. The result after selecting and assembling all the counted correct atoms is two complete cells. His second "division" system is called "meiosis" in which He starts with one cell and finishes His assembly work with four cells called 'gametes' which are used for reproduction.

"Meiosis" is the name given to the work of producing the egg and the sperm cells which, when combined, are further constructed into a new organism that is a blend of the mother's and father's features.

Why do we call God a "Him" and why do we think He is *superintelligent*? Easy questions and easy answers: In 2016, the three Nobel Prize Winners in Chemistry (J.P. Sauvage, Sir J.F. Stoddart, and B.L. Feringa) were awarded this prestigious prize for their work over a 33-year period to develop some tiny molecular machines. The best they could construct were far simpler than the simplest molecular machines built daily for our new cells. What their work shows us is that even with mankind's vast accumulation of scientific knowledge and highly sophisticated equipment, we do not have anywhere near enough intelligence, skill, or ability to build even the simplest molecular machines for our cells. This establishes that "superintelligence" (far above the human level) is essential to build living molecular machines. The reason this entity is called "He" and "Him" is that the only omniscient being known to mankind (i.e., God) is referred to as both "Father" and "Son" in His Word, the Holy Bible. He is known by our governments and most of our citizens as "God," as in "One Nation Under God," "In God We Trust," "God Save The King," "God Keep Our Land Glorious and Free," the God of Thanksgiving Day, Christmas, and Easter -- *that* God.

It is interesting to note that in the Bible, He describes one of the most valuable things anyone can acquire -- Wisdom -- as "She" and "Her." (See Proverbs 8:1-3; 9:1).

These 2016 Nobel Prize winners also have clearly verified for us, probably unintentionally, that anything having <u>no</u> intelligence (like Darwin's theoretical evolution) is factually out of the running as the cause and sustainer of life.

We can logically conclude that this all-knowing entity called God, is the only one who could build the original cells for each species, as well as all cells since.

Persons, including teachers and college professors, who have been taught that intelligence is not required to create life because evolution can do it, must carefully consider the evidence presented in this book, that is, if they desire to teach **truth** and accuracy.

If someone claims that "natural mechanisms" can design and construct complex molecular machines, such as mitochondria and proteins for our cells, they must explain how these "natural mechanisms" are constructed first containing far more intelligence and better equipment than our Nobel Prize winners possessed.

Scientists called "cytologists" who study cells know of over 40 different types of molecular machines constructed for our over 200 different cell types. These include skin cells, muscle cells, nerve cells, retina cells to enable us to see, smell cells to smell, heart cells to pump our blood, brain cells to think, and the 200+ other cell types.

As nano-observers inside Johnny's forefinger, let's watch God do His brilliant and careful works in building just one of the trillions of new cells for Johnny.

God has already constructed the capillary network (small blood vessels) to carry the required building supplies from Johnny's digestive system, lungs, and liver to this specific cell construction site. He has also constructed the wiring necessary to achieve muscle control, pain-warning, and other sensory messages to Johnny's brain, plus intercellular communication and co-ordination systems. Next, the decision has to be made as to what specific cell type to construct next. Should it be a muscle cell? A skin cell? A nerve cell? A fat cell? A fingernail or bone cell? Actually, the builder (God) has already decided what type of cell is needed to be built here. In this case it is a skin cell.

As the atoms for constructing this cell are moving rapidly inside the capillary, and the blood carrying about 60 kinds of atoms is under pressure, He has to construct a tiny controllable opening at the proper place on the capillary. The control allows only the re-quired atoms to be transferred into the cell construction site which starts within an adjacent cell, but, at the same time, not permit the blood, which is under pressure, to flood the construction site.

One reason God begins building a new cell within an adjacent cell is to extend the existing communication wiring from the brain into the new cell for pain and muscle response. He also builds the cells to achieve intercellular communication to help coordinate the work of the cells in that area. As a result, large groups of cells called tissues, work as a unit, cooperating to produce a functional system.

The cell parts that must be constructed include 'lipids' and proteins for assembling the outer layer of the cell membrane using the correctly counted numbers of the proper elemental atoms.

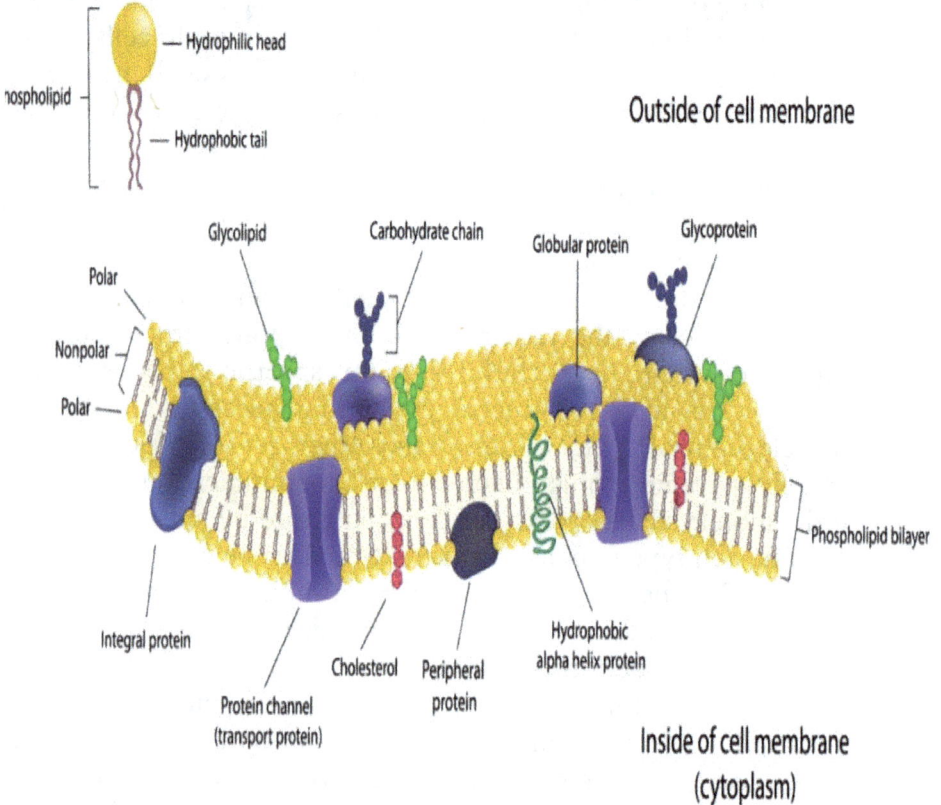

Kallayanee Naloka / Shutterstock

This plan for just the outer membrane of the new cell helps us glean the complexity of the cell construction project. This is the "easy" part compared to building the complex molecular machinery that must be constructed inside the cell membrane.

Johnny's cell parts (and ours) have to be constructed very carefully. For example, the 20 amino acids needed as parts for the construction of human cells, must be assembled with the same foundational group of four atoms: $H_4 N_1 C_2 O_2$ then:

For Glycine the formula is $H_5 N_1 C_2 O_2$
For Alanine " " " $H_7 N_1 C_3 O_2$
For Valine " " " $H_{11} N_1 C_5 O_2$

and so on for all of the other 17 amino acids required for life.

Notice how accurately the atoms must be selected from our blood stream which picks them up from our digestive system, lungs, and liver. The correct atom types must be selected from among the many types available in the adjacent blood vessel, then carefully counted, and precisely assembled to construct each amino acid.

The next chapter shows the details for assembling the four bases for our DNA which guides our cells' functions.

Scientists have been trying for over seventy years to produce a living cell from elements and cannot come anywhere close. Even with our vast accumulation of scientific knowledge and sophisticated equipment we just do not have enough intelligence.

The essential change for the science community to accept regarding the construction of living cells for all life, including humans, is this: the physical work of finding, sorting, selecting, counting, and precisely assembling in sequence the correct numbers of the correct atoms for every cell part for every living cell, can only be performed by a superintelligent being.

There is only one such entity known to mankind. Our governments and the majority of our thinking citizens call this entity, "our Creator, God" as in, "We hold these truths to be self-evident, that all men are **created** equal, that they are endowed by **their Creator** with certain unalienable Rights,....",[1] "one nation under **God**,"[2] "In **God** We Trust"[3] - *that* **God**. (See Chapters 10-13).

Our students have the "unalienable right" to be taught why God is so highly recognized by their governments. Now the newly developed life science of "atomic biology" provides scientific reasons.

After our Creator completes constructing the complex outer membrane for Johnny's skin cell, He must construct the inner parts of the cell that, when completed, look something like this:

ANATOMY OF A CELL

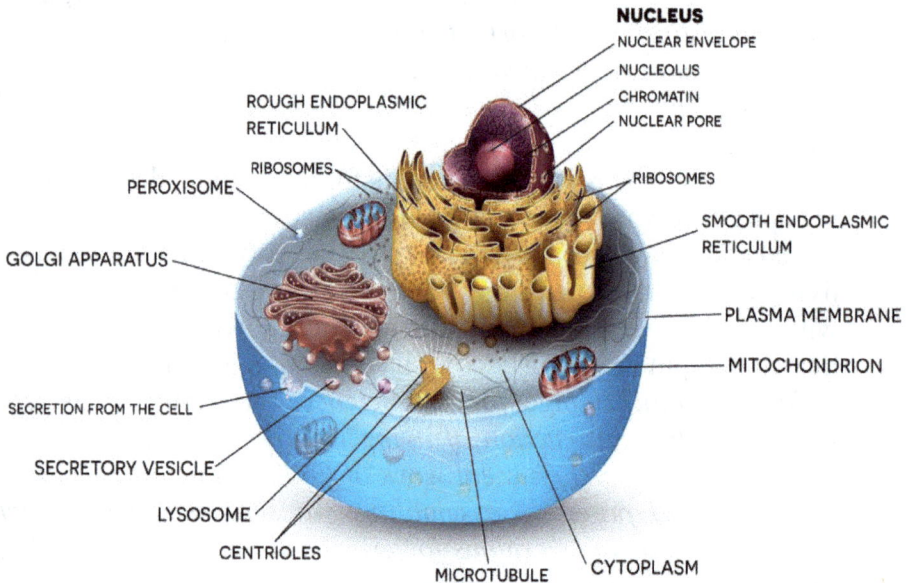

NUCLEUS
- NUCLEAR ENVELOPE
- NUCLEOLUS
- CHROMATIN
- NUCLEAR PORE

ROUGH ENDOPLASMIC RETICULUM

RIBOSOMES

PEROXISOME

RIBOSOMES

SMOOTH ENDOPLASMIC RETICULUM

GOLGI APPARATUS

PLASMA MEMBRANE

MITOCHONDRION

SECRETION FROM THE CELL

SECRETORY VESICLE

LYSOSOME

CENTRIOLES

MICROTUBULE

CYTOPLASM

Tefi / Shutterstock

Above is a diagram of a "eukaryotic" cell which is a much more complex cell than a prokaryotic cell such as a bacterium, however, even bacterial cells are amazingly complex. Eukaryotic cells are the building blocks for all multicellular organisms. They contain membrane-bound organelles not used in prokaryotic cells.

Other parts not shown include the DNA helix which is about two meters long with about six billion parts precisely arranged.

Another major point is that the atoms Johnny's cells are made of do not have "Life" individually. God provides their electrons with a constant and controlled supply of energy for their perpetual

30

motion, but this motion is not "Life". This essential ingredient called *"the breath of life"* must be added to each new cell for life to exist. When it is removed, the cell can no longer live or function.

In a child, the first cells began with the union of a mother's egg cell with a father's sperm cell which form a **zygote.** This first united cell contains **chromosomes** that contain the plan for its traits, including hair-color, eye-color, and skin-color, gender, and adult height, that come partly from the mother and partly from the father. This information and some of the DNA is duplicated in most of the other cells in the child, up to adulthood. This is how features of the parents are designed for the child.

After the two-cell union forms the zygote, a morula is constructed which is a solid spherical-shaped ball of 16 cells. God builds these cells by duplicating some of the information in the zygote and precisely assembling more selected and correctly counted atoms from the mother to build the complete 16 new cells in the morula.

Then in about five days after egg cell fertilization occurs, the morula is developed into a **blastocyst**.

This careful work is how our Creator began constructing each one of us.

From here on, new cell types have to be constructed in proper sequence to make the required blood cells, bone cells, heart cells, brain cells, skull, liver, and so on, each one at the right place and time. These require ultrasmart choices, decisions, atom selections, counting, and correct assembly of the parts.

By day 22, the brain will be sufficiently developed, along with the skull, limbs, skeleton, blood vessels, blood cells, and a beating heart to pump the blood with all the nutrient atoms needed for this little person to begin functioning.

God must continue the body construction to adulthood, building about 100 trillion cells of over 200 different types, most of which contain a DNA molecule with about three billion base pairs programmed to provide function instructions. A few cell types, called enucleated cells, including blood and eye lens cells, discard their DNA. Up to 40 different molecular machines called "organelles", are constructed within each cell. The divine "breath of life" must be installed into every cell, as no cell can function without it.

Speculation about how cells function was unsuccessful until the invention of the microscope in the 1600s. Englishman Robert Hooke, researching cork cells and other plant tissues in 1665, used the term "cell" because the cellulose walls of dead cork cells reminded him of the monastery cells occupied by Christian monks. So complex is the cell that it has taken scientists over 300 years to understand how it works. We are still learning new details about its design, construction, and function today.

Much was unknown about atoms, molecules, cells, and life, in Darwin's time. He admitted a number of ways exist that his theory could "absolutely break down." *The fact today is, now that we understand the cell and its superb design and complex construction, his theory of evolution has 'absolutely broken down.'*

After many decades of study, some evolutionists, as well as most former evolutionists, agree that the concept of an original reproducing cell (called "the common ancestor") coming to life by chance, is logically impossible.

Now we know there was no "common ancestor" as Darwin postulated, but there is a common designer and builder.

According to Dr. Stephen C. Meyer of the Discovery Institute, the *simplest* known cell today, a bacterium, requires a whopping 482 proteins and 562,000 DNA bases for it to function. [4]

Knowing how precisely assembled each amino acid, protein, and DNA base has to be constructed, puts the probability of even this simplest known living cell just happening by time, chance, mutations, and evolution, into the zero zone.

Scientists are still learning more about the phenomenal complexities essential for constructing the over 40 different molecular machines to perform our cells' various functions. For example, an average-sized DNA strand requires about 6,000,000,000 (six billion) bases (i.e. arranged as three billion base pairs) to be assembled in a precise sequence like words in a book to serve as the operating instructions for an average cell.

The essentiality of ultra-intelligent works in constructing our highly complex cell parts, is illustrated by the fact that, as noted earlier, three of the brightest scientific minds on the planet, the 2016 Nobel Prize winners in Chemistry, equipped with the most sophisticated equipment ever developed for constructing molecular machines from atoms, could not come anywhere close to constructing even the simplest molecular machines that we require to carry out our many essential cell functions. *Therefore, "evolution", having no intelligence to use, is totally disqualified as the cause of Life. Life can only come through the super-intelligent and careful work of our Creator, God.*

Our Molecular Machines	Their Function(s)
Adaptive Immune System	Helps our body fight off germs
Aminoacyl-tRNA Synthetases	Helps enzymes making proteins
Antibodies	Fight germs (pathogens)
ATP Synthase	Charges our body's "batteries"
Bacterial Flagella	Transporters in our body fluids
Blood-clotting Cascade	Prevents most hemorrhaging
Calcium Pump	Moves calcium into our cells

A few of the many other complex cell parts required for human life include: ribosome, spliceosome, myosin, kinesin, tim/tom systems, cytochrome C oxidase, proteasome, cohesin, condensin, clpX, immunological synapse, glideosome, kex2, hsp70, hsp60, protein kinase C, secYEG preprotein translocation channel, hemoglobin, T4 DNA packaging motor, smc5smc6, cytoplasmic dynien, mitotic spindle machine, DNA polymerase, RNA polymerase, kinetochore, MRX complex, apoptosome/caspase, type III secretory system, type II secretion apparatus, helicase/topoisomerase machine, RNA degradasome, photosynthetic system, and eukaryotic cilia.

(See also Chapter 5: *Our Incredible Molecular Machines,* especially pages 71-72).

All of this phenomenal construction work is performed for Johnny and every one of us every second of every day at no charge.

God reliably and continuously constructs, sustains, maintains, repairs, and replaces our cells for us.

Would you agree that, at the very least, He does deserve our gratitude?

Applications for Life

1. What kind of entity is needed to construct new cells and what do we call this being? _____

_____

2. What group showed that mankind does not have enough intelligence to construct living cell parts? _____

_____

3. How did they show that a superintelligent being is necessary to build molecular machines for our cells?

_____

_____

_____

4. What does the need for intelligence in building cell parts and cells show about Darwin's evolution? _____

_____

_____

5. What are three of the areas where God is part of our national government? _____

_____

6. How can you explain the problem when someone claims that "natural mechanisms" build our cell parts and cells for us?

_____

_____

_____

_____

7. How many different types of molecular machines are required for the operating functions of our many different cells? _____

8. How many different types of cells do we have? _____

9. Name three parts of a cell membrane.

_____

_____

10. How many bases are in the simplest cell known today?

_____

11. How many proteins are in the simplest cell known today?

_____

12. How many bases have to be physically placed in correct sequence to construct an average-sized molecular strand of DNA.

_____

References and Notes:

[1] U.S. Declaration of Independence.

[2] U.S. Pledge of Allegiance.

[3] On U.S. currency and public buildings.

[4] Meyer, Stephen C., *Signature in the Cell,* Harper Collins, New York, NY, 2009, p. 201.

Chapter 3
Our Phenomenal DNA and RNA

What is DNA ?

DNA, which stands for deoxyribonucleic acid, is crucial in helping cells perform their multitudes of amazing functions.

The main components of the DNA code include 4 bases:
Adenine - chemical formula $C_5 H_5 N_5$
Guanine -   "   " $C_5 H_5 N_5 O_1$
Cytosine -   "   " $C_4 H_5 N_3 O_1$
Thymine -   "   " $C_5 H_6 N_2 O_2$

Notice how similar the formulae are for these bases. As each one is being constructed for us using atoms from our digestive system via our bloodstreams, it is critical that the builder be absolutely precise with the design and in the selection, counting, and placement of the correct numbers of the correct atoms, as well as fastening the right bases in the proper sequences in programming our DNA for the various required functions in our cells. What great intelligence, dexterity, and care this requires.

Some people credit chemical reactions for the assembly of cells and entities, but with a little thought we can see that simply having C, H, N, and O hook up by chemical attraction would not make the life-giving choices and decisions for the precise numbers of each elemental atom to choose, count, and fasten per base. If the numbers of any of the atoms for any of these bases were not precisely correct, the whole DNA program would be corrupt causing a crash in the operation of the cell.

DNA is a super-sized strand of molecules (sometimes called a macromolecule) reaching up to two meters in length in a single cell according to Bruce Alberts and his co-authors in *Molecular Biology of the Cell*, Fourth Edition.[1] Almost all of our trillions of microscopic cells have an enormous DNA strand built into each one. The whole strand is wrapped into either the nucleus or the cytoplasm in each cell.

DNA macromolecules are the most spectacular of all the machines constructed in our cells. Approximately 3,000,000,000 (three billion) base pairs must be assembled within most of our 80 trillion cells that require DNA, using the right numbers of the correct types of atoms. The arrangement sequence is a huge, programmed code outlining our genetic information, heredity, a communication system, and instructions to help operate and maintain the cell. Its living computer software program has immense intelligent coding of our heredity from both parents (based on 23 chromosomes from our mother's egg and 23 chromosomes from our father's sperm). The programming also produces our individuality and assists with the various specific functions for which each cell is designed and amazingly built of atoms.

Microsoft founder, Bill Gates, stated, "Human DNA is like a computer program but far, far more advanced than any software we've ever created." [2]

Scientist I.L. Cohen said, *"At that moment, when the RNA/DNA system became understood, the debate between Evolutionists and Creationists should have come to a screeching halt."* [3] He is rightfully noting that when the enormous complexity of RNA and DNA programming was discovered, the theory of evolution, should have been dropped because evolution does not possess intelligence to program DNA.

All functional coding systems were *constructed* by an intelligent builder, and we know of no intelligent coding that is *improved* without intelligent help. The tendency to deteriorate (the second law of thermodynamics) typically results when coding changes are not guided by intelligence. This applies to the immense coding in DNA as well.

Parts of our personal DNA strands (about 1%) are unique for each one of us. This feature helps authorities identify a person without consciousness or identification, who is hurt, involved in a crime, or must be cleared for security purposes.

Other parts of these same DNA strands (roughly the other 99%) are virtually identical to our eight+ billion neighbors. These genes are involved in coding for our eyesight, hearing, tasting, brain, liver and nerve cells, plus the other 200+ types of cells, that govern the required functions that are the same for all humans.

Further differences are made in some of the cells for males and females. These differences are primarily for producing and raising children.

Each of our approximately 100 trillion cells is more complex than an entire city. Online sites display comparisons between functioning parts of a city to functioning parts of our cells. Rough analogies portrayed often consist of the following examples:

Cell Nucleus – The City Hall which coordinates the city's necessary functions;

Nuclear Membrane – The City Hall fence with security guards;

Mitochondria – The power plants which generate controlled energy for cell operation and highly-regulated body temperature;

Cell Membrane – The city border;

Cell Wall – A city wall with security guards;

Endoplasmic Reticulum – a manufacturing/assembly plant;

DNA – Extensive detailed plans for building and running the city;

Nucleolus – A control center that regulates many city functions;

RNA – Plan copies for use around the city;

Chromosomes – Instructions from the founders;

Ribosomes – Building materials assembly;

Proteins – Workers;

Vacuole – Water tower;

Cytoplasm – Atmosphere;

Protoplasm – Moisture in the atmosphere;

Golgi Apparatus – Post office;

Lysosomes – Recyclers and waste disposers.

All these types of functions and more are necessary for running a cell. For a city there must be a huge amount of intelligent planning, construction, servicing, maintenance, repair work, security, and fire department. So it is with each of our cells.

While cities generally require decades to design and construct, our cells are built in a matter of minutes or hours. This work began as soon as we were conceived.

The construction of our cities takes an enormous amount of human intelligence, knowledge, dexterity, skills, and physical work. The construction of our cells requires an even greater amount of, knowledge, dexterity, construction skills, and physical work, plus lightning speed, and greater accuracy.

The amount of information programmed into the DNA in each of our cells is typically estimated as enough to fill more than a thousand sets of encyclopedias; or, if printed out in 12-point font, the printed line of information would reach from the North Pole to the Equator. These rough examples are commonly used by scientists to give us a picture that shows the amount of intelligent coding in our DNA is gigantic.

The potential technological benefits of mimicking the applications of DNA technology is large. For example, George Church and Sri Kosuri at Harvard University, and a group headed by Nick Goldman at the European Bioinformatics Institute, Cambridge, England have developed synthesized, non-living DNA for super-sized storage of digital information. The storage capacity-to-size ratio of DNA saves a dramatic amount of space and is a safer way to ensure data accuracy in long-term storage. The main shortcoming is that the process remains costly.

Our personal DNA is live, active, functional, and repaired if damaged. It is a life-supporting marvel, designed and built by our caring Creator, along with the rest of our body, mind, and spirit.

Below is an image of the shape of a segment of the molecule strand that holds information within most of our cells. These graphic images of a DNA helix are expanded thousands of times larger than real life-size to allow us to visualize them.

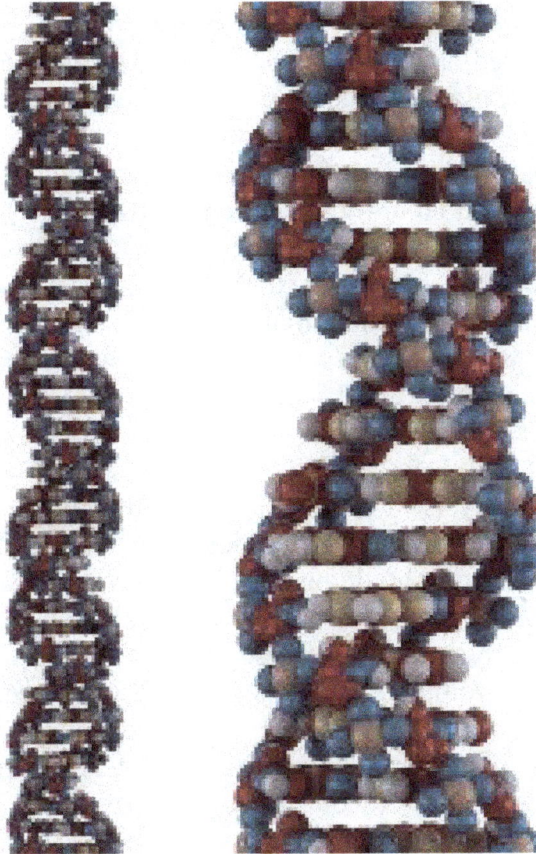

Mopic/Shutterstock.com

Our amazing DNA is designed with double helixes precisely built primarily of specially designed proteins. These proteins require enormous intelligent programming at lightning speed, especially in our cells that have a lifespan of only a few days. This process goes far beyond the parameters of possibility for any unguided process.

It would be interesting to estimate the number of computer programmers required to program the functional coding for just one cell's DNA in four days, for example. Of course, they would have to *know* the exact coding needed and how to assemble the right numbers of the required bases before beginning.

These factors point to the immense amount of brilliant physical work required to precisely place and fasten all the correct numbers of the required atoms, by a phenomenally intelligent, dexterous, and caring entity. In the English language, we call this entity "God".

We must consume the food types that provide sufficient atoms of each required 60 or more element kinds for God to build all of our body's cell parts.

The sooner we investigate the atomic needs of each type of our cells, plus the atomic content of fruits, vegetables, meats, and fish, the sooner we can match our recommended foods to our body's requirements. Some food items might lack some of their normal elements if the soil they were grown in lacked some of those elements.

Atomic analysis of field soil content, conducted to match the atomic requirements of our various food items, will reveal what fertilizer elements should be added to the soil for each crop.

On a topic related to our DNA, we must recognize that our cells do not just replicate themselves. What would happen if the first cell in our development were a toe cell? If cells only replicated themselves, then would we each become one big toe? The answer is obvious. Each new cell of chosen different types, has to be constructed carefully by our Creator.

Each of the 200+ different types of cells required to produce the human body has a different design, uses different elements, structures, different DNA and RNA for different functions.

With all of this remarkably detailed, wondrous work, carefully and awesomely built and programmed into our DNA, God clearly deserves our appreciation.

What is RNA? RNA stands for ribonucleic acid. It is another macromolecule like DNA that is essential for the functioning of cells in all known forms of life.

RNA is also composed of four bases: Adenine, Guanine, Cytosine, but the Thymine ($C_5 H_6 N_2 O_2$) is replaced by Uracil -

chemical formula $C_4 H_4 N_2 O_2$ (again having a very similar but purposefully different chemical formula requiring ultrasmart and careful assembly.

Molecular biology has shown that the flow of genetic inform-ation is from our DNA through our RNA to the various "workhorses" (molecular machines) in our cells. As mentioned, the information has to be programmed into our various cells' DNA.

Since different cells have different functions, so the DNA programming has to be slightly different from cell-type to cell-type; it is not just copied.

In the control of the genes, some are repressed and activated, and up-regulated or down-regulated. Also, cell parts have different jobs to do within each cell, and the RNA molecules communicate the various work instructions to the various cellular molecular machines.

rRNA is a structural component of ribosomes which are molecular machines that guide the production of proteins within the cell from the RNA blueprints. Some RNA molecules can also act as enzymes called ribozymes.

Decisions and Choices

This all leads to the following crucial question: for those who believe that God designed and built the amazing biological systems for humans into Adam and Eve and has never intervened in our construction, sustenance, maintenance, or repair since, how do we account for all the superintelligent decisions, choices, and physical works necessary to construct any part of us. For example, deciding when to switch from assembling a blood vessel's outer membrane cell to a muscle cell, a nerve cell, or an eye-part cell right beside the vessel membrane cell?

In the human body, there are about 60 different elements used to make all the various parts for all our 200+ types of cells. There are virtually countless decisions and choices to make just in selecting and counting the correct atoms needed to make all the various molecules for all the various parts of our various cells.

Assembling and programming the DNA macromolecule in *just one* of our skin cells for example, knowing that this contains the equivalent amount of information of roughly 1000 sets of encyclopedias, is mind-boggling. Think of the number of choices and decisions necessary for selecting and precisely assembling the correct numbers of the required atoms from our blood stream for that one part of that one skin cell. Then making the decisions and choices necessary for assembling the many other different molecular machines for that one skin cell; then switching to building a muscle cell right next to the skin cell with a totally different structure and function.

It is really all these decisions, choices, and physical works with atoms that rule out everything but a superintelligent being for creating living cells and biological creatures like us.

We, and our governments call this brilliant and caring entity our "Creator God." "Thanksgiving Day" is a national day of appreciation for His phenomenal work, sacrifice, provision, and care for us.

Applications for Life:

1. For the DNA bases, what four chemical elements are carefully assembled for us to live?

   _____

   _____

2. About how many pairs of these bases must be assembled in precise sequence for each DNA macromolecule in each of our nucleated cells? _____

3. What great software company boss admitted that, "Human DNA is like a computer program but far, far more advanced than any software we've ever created."? _____

4. Who is the only one who can create our DNA by selecting, counting, and assembling atoms in the right sequence for each of our cells? _____

5. To what large common thing is a human cell often compared?

_____

References and Notes:

[1] "The Structure and Function of DNA," *Molecular Biology of the Cell*, Fourth Edition, National Center for Biotechnology Information, Bethesda, MA, www.ncbi.nlm.nih.gov/books/NBK26821/, accessed July 3, 2014.

[2] Gates, Bill, Nathan Myhrvold, and Peter Rinearson, *The Road Ahead: Completely Revised and Up-To-Date,* Penguin Books, New York, NY, 1996, p. 228.

[3] Cohen, I. L., *Darwin Was Wrong: A Study in Probabilities,* Research Publications, New York, NY, 1984, p. 5.

Chapter 4
Our Amazing Systems and Senses

As we have established from grade school science, every material object is made of atoms. This includes all parts of our body. Where do the atoms for building us come from? From the food we consume and air we breathe. In our beginning, most of the required atoms came to us through our umbilical cord attached to our mother's womb and blood system.

And where do those atoms for our food and oxygen come from? From the soil of gardens, fields, and orchards, and the fresh air from plants that take in carbon dioxide and produce fresh oxygen. Then what happens after we have eaten and breathed in these atoms from our food and air?

The atoms from our digestive system and lungs are delivered by our blood system to all parts of our body for use in repairing cells or assembling new cells where needed in our tissues, organs, bloodstream, nerves, brain, limbs, and the rest of our 200+ cell types.

All of this activity takes a phenomenal amount of designing, planning, and physical work – 24/7 – for our entire life.

This is the result of the enormous loving care for us by our awesome Creator.

People who have figured out that God loves them, even if they did not know these details, receive a special benefit through their relationship with their Creator. Showing personal appreciation for God's work and care for all of us is a form of devotion, but the rest of this knowledge is pure science.

The detailed construction and functions of *each one* of our systems and senses could fill a large encyclopedia which this book is not, so we are going to provide a brief overview of each marvelous one.

OUR BODY SYSTEMS

1. Our Digestion System

After we consume food (or medicine) and breathe in air, the huge task of sorting atoms begins in our digestive system and lungs.

The work of breaking our food down into smaller and smaller pieces begins in our mouth. Chewing our food properly helps to mix the digestive juices in our mouth with our food to begin digestion.

The next step of further breaking down our food into smaller pieces is performed in our stomach where strong digestive juices such as hydrochloric acid are produced.

Then the atoms have to be absorbed into our bloodstream for delivery to all parts of our body.

God has to select the needed numbers of the correct atoms from our food to construct new cells for us to grow when we are young and to replace worn-out or damaged cells at any age. He also has to deliver certain atoms from our food to all our cells for their energy supply, sustenance, maintenance, and repair.

Some cells need repairing because of damage by cuts, scrapes or other abuse. Many are damaged to the degree that they need replacing. Our red blood cells wear out after about 120 days of absorbing and delivering oxygen to the cells and removing carbon dioxide. For an average-size adult male (based on a 70-kilogram or 154-pound male), about 2,300,000 new red blood cells (RBCs) must be built and delivered into his bloodstream *every second* of every day.[1] (You can relate these numbers to your own weight).

Then they are delivered into the bloodstream, and the old ones removed and partially recycled or delivered to our waste system.

This requires handling more atoms to replace our worn-out RBCs. More food has to be constructed including the roots, leaves, and skins which are thrown away. Therefore, this brings the total to more than 12,800 quadrillion atoms per second that must be properly assembled for the replacement of just red blood cells for a 150-pounder.

We have another roughly 80,000,000,000,000 (80 trillion) cells that also must be maintained, repaired, and replaced to keep us alive and healthy. These mind-boggling numbers indicate how much each one of us is continuously cared for by our Creator.

Of course, *we also* have to take some responsibility for our health and well-being. We are given the freedom to choose what we put into our mouth or inhale. We require a balance of healthful foods and beverages.

We need to avoid substances that abuse our body. We shouldn't expect to stay healthy by smoking, drinking excessive alcohol, using addictive drugs, and eating junk food. God makes the best foods for us and we should focus on consuming those foods.

Reasonable exercise helps our digestive process as well as our muscle capacity, circulation, energy supply, attitude, and overall wellness. Common sense, balanced physical activity, and self-care all play a major role in our quality and enjoyment of life.

2. Our Respiratory System

The quality of what we inhale is also important to our health because some of the atoms God needs to use for building, sustaining, maintaining, and repairing our body, come from the air we breathe.

Unfortunately, many of the air pollutants in our cities adversely affect the quality of the air we breathe. Inhaling cigarette smoke and poisons like cocaine and other drugs will ruin our health over time. This brings suffering of one kind or another.

As we are told repeatedly, exercise and fresh air are important for our health. The deep breathing brought on by exercising increases our crucial oxygen supply and helps eliminate the toxins in our body. Part of God's great design and physical work for our lives is to use the carbon-dioxide we exhale for the construction of trees and plants. These plants in turn, produce oxygen which God then uses for our construction, sustenance, maintenance, and repair.

It is important to understand that our governments cannot solve all of our problems, and God won't either. They should not be expected to do so. We are blessed with many free choices but we need to use wisdom in choosing the way we manage our lives; otherwise we will suffer from unnecessary troubles. Our choices produce consequences for us.

It is up to us to help take care of ourselves, our nation, and our allies.

3. Our Blood System

As mentioned, God has to perform an enormous amount of work for us just to replace our worn-out red blood cells. Sorting, selecting, grasping, precisely placing and fastening more than 4900 quadrillion atoms per second for an average person, just to build our replacement red blood cells, goes far beyond the parameters of possibility for any unguided process like evolution.

Our blood system has many crucial jobs to perform including, but not limited to:

1. Collecting oxygen from the air we breathe into our lungs and transporting it to every cell;

2. Delivering the carbon dioxide our cells exhaust as waste back to our lungs to be exhaled;

3. Gathering many kinds of atoms from our digestive systems and delivering them as nutrients to each of our other cells for their energy, nourishment, maintenance, and repair;

4. Delivering damaged or worn-out cell parts to our waste system for disposal;

5. Helping to regulate our body temperature which is crucial to maintain within very small variation. Just a few degrees deviation in either direction can be lethal;

6. Delivering God-designed and built healing molecules to the wounded areas of our body;

7. Helping our immune system to fight invasive pathogens and viruses;

8. Disposing of these foreign invaders to our waste system;

9. Delivering of atoms from pharmaceuticals taken to places within us where they are required to help fight colds, headaches, and other illnesses;

10. Blood-clotting to prevent hemorrhages; and more.

4. Our Excretory System

After our digestive system has broken down our foods into small parts, and God has sorted, selected, grasped, and taken all of the right atoms He needs to work with for our cell sustenance, maintenance, repair, and replacement, He leaves the unneeded atoms in our bloodstream for delivery to our waste system for elimination.

Disposing of our waste is another crucial part of our life systems. Additional waste includes worn-out cells, destroyed pathogens, liquid wastes, toxins, and so on. This is another marvelous part of the design, construction, and operation of our body.

Regular eliminations of toxic wastes are crucial for our health.

5. Our Nervous System

This is another phenomenal part that God builds into us to aid our body functions.

Nerves are the amazing hard-wiring for all the electrical messaging necessary for our brain and muscle functions, eyesight, hearing, touching, tasting, smelling, and the operation of our conscious and subconscious activities.

According to scientists Van Wedeen and L.L. Wald, each human brain contains approximately *100,000 miles (160,000 kilometers)* of nerve fibers.[2]

Using separate nerve-fiber lines, God also connects all of the following to our brain:
- every one of our muscles;
- all parts of our speech system;
- every skin-cell sensor for our sense of touch and pain-warning;
- all parts of our other senses, including our eyesight, taste, smell, and hearing;
- all our organs for their functioning;
- and, of course, the fantastic communications and function systems within our brain itself.

God also builds more spectacular messaging systems into most of our 100 trillion cells to help guide all of the amazing work that goes on in each cell. Just reading and responding to the functional instructions within the DNA to guide the work in each cell, boggles one's mind.

The amazing complexity constructed into each little part of our body is virtually overwhelming. Wouldn't you agree?

6. Our Immune System

Here is another amazing system that God has designed and built into each of us. Because we are not able to keep perfectly clean, and both helpful and harmful bacteria are all around us, He has created in us an internal system to combat the harmful bacteria, and viruses. We can strengthen this system against some pathogens by using vaccinations.

Actually, living in a non-sterile environment having some dust, dirt, and germs functions like vaccination, protecting us in the future. The other help is to make sure that we eat healthful foods and beverages, get fresh air, and exercise. These take a little planning and willpower but are probably the best investments we will ever make for our body.

7. Our Reproductive System

This is the most phenomenal and spectacular system of all because this is used by our Creator to build all our magnificent parts, systems, and senses. Then He connects them all with blood vessels and nerves and covers them with skin to make this fantastic, living machine in which we live called the human body.

The marvelous work of building each one of us began when our mother was born. At that time God had constructed about 400,000 egg cells into her little ovaries for future use.[3] Although she lost one or more eggs with each menstrual cycle, one of the remainders was available for fertilization and the beginning of our life.

These egg cells were constantly sustained with nourishment and maintained in good condition so that one of them could provide its special role in our assembly. The job of that one special egg cell was to provide about half the design features for the construction of all our regular parts and unique features, looks, and traits when our time came to be created.

When the time came for our mother to be able to bear children, God would send one or more of these egg cells from their storage area in her ovaries, down towards her baby construction site – her womb – in preparation for possible fertilization which would begin the baby construction process.

Normally, one egg cell would be released from our mother's ovaries every month. If no fertilization occurred within a few days, the egg cell would be flushed out of her womb along with some special blood lining that was in her uterus to support the possible baby construction process.

This monthly cycle continued until it was our time to be created. When our month to be conceived finally came, it was time for our father to get involved.

He had to provide a fertilizer cell, called a sperm cell, to unite with our mother's egg cell. This was the easy part for him; then he was supposed to support, and if he was an honorable man, he *did* support his wife and the family members he helped to produce.

Once the mother's egg cell and father's sperm cell united, our Creator began the amazing task of building us from the "dust" with His phenomenal two-step process - with atoms from the soil, he made our foods and from atoms in our foods, He made our cells. He constructed our unique features in accordance with the plans that were built into the original egg cell and sperm cell.

All the food atoms not needed for building us plus sustaining, maintaining, and repairing or replacing our mother's cells, were disposed of through her waste system.

God generally takes about nine months to build a human baby. There is currently a great video found on YouTube by searching "Alexander Tsiaris Conception to Birth – Visualized" from medical image maker Alexander Tsiaras at a TED Talks INK conference. Hopefully it is still showing as you read this passage. The phenomenal sequence of construction from the fertilization of an egg to the birth of a baby normally follows these steps:

- **Day 1:** The mother's egg is released from one of her two ovaries and is captured by one of her two oviducts.

- Shortly after the egg enters the oviduct, it may be met with a sperm. The egg is designed with complex sensors and mechanisms to allow generally only one sperm, and nothing other than human sperm, to enter the egg.
- The fertilized egg is moved down the oviduct and begins to divide and be constructed into two cells. If the two cells separate and live, identical twins will begin to be constructed. If two eggs happen to be fertilized by separate sperm, non-identical twins will begin to be constructed. For our purpose, we will stay with the construction of a single child. This could be us.

- **Day 6:** The fertilized egg cell is fastened to the wall of our mother's womb with filtered access to nutrient atoms from our mother's blood vessels.

- **Day 25:** An amazing amount of physical work has been performed, including the gathering of the needed numbers of the correct atoms from the nutrients delivered by our mother's blood stream from the digesting food in her intestines to the uterus (womb). The selection, counting, grasping, precise placement, and fastening of the counted numbers of the correct atoms were used to construct us as an embryo to the point of having a recognizable head, spine, and heart which is beating by this day.

Day 56: The all-wise entity we call God has already assembled all of our organs to an early stage. From there on He had to complete our construction which involved the precise assembly of approximately 4.2 trillion cells. He made collagen tissue, which is stronger than steel by relative weight, to hold us as a fetus with our marvelous parts all together in their proper place.

Almost all of our cells under construction had their own DNA instructions built into them and programmed with phenomenal amounts of information (see Chapter 3 for more about our DNA).

Of course, all the atoms used for building the cells have no life of their own, therefore, God's crucial "breath-of-life" had to be added to make each cell live and function.

There had to be a skin made for us to hold everything together and, incidentally, our skin is the largest organ of our body.

Within this skin, God had to build for us a brain, a heart, blood, and blood vessels within about the first three weeks of our construction timeline. Then He continued to build a liver, kidneys, stomach, intestines, pancreas, gall bladder, eyes, ears, nose mouth, hair, arms, hands, legs, feet, fingernails, toenails, skeleton, muscles, lungs, nerves, wiring, and the rest of our body parts. In addition, He had to program our DNA in almost all of our cells so that everything functions properly together. He also had to make several organs that are different for girls and boys.

What an enormous amount of beautiful, phenomenal, superintelligent effort He put into designing and building each one of us. What wonderful, careful works He provided and continues to provide to us in making our foods and reassembling our food atoms into our new cells for our growth, maintenance, and repair every second of every day.

An average-sized human baby human weighs about 7 pounds (3.2 kg) at birth, and then over the next twenty years, grows to become an adult. An average male is about 154 pounds (70 kg). This is about 22 times the size of the little baby at birth.

To build an adult of this size, God has to construct about 100 trillion (100,000,000,000,000) cells compared to the approximately 5 trillion (5,000,000,000,000) cells when we were born. As He builds us He has to provide His breath-of-life to each cell as He completes it.

He takes about nine months working quickly and brilliantly – twenty-four hours a day – to build each one of us to the point of birth. He initially got the atoms from our mother's womb until He had built our umbilical cord, which He then attached from our little body to the special blood vessels in our mother's womb.

Incidentally, as God has to begin building each baby with a sperm and an egg, it would not have been difficult for Him to build both of these in the Virgin Mary's womb.

OUR MARVELOUS SENSES

1. Our Sense of Sight

What a fantastic invention this is, and what a phenomenally intelligent construction project.

Our eyes are the most valuable and intricate of all our senses. Blind people adjust to life and heighten other senses including hearing and touch, but they miss so much that we with vision take for granted. Being able to see the world around us is of enormous value, helping to make our life interesting, safe, and enjoyable.

These small round organs have many parts, all of which are responsible for sight, protection, maintenance, and clarity. People are sometimes born with different-shaped eyes that can distort vision but this can now be corrected by man-made lenses or surgeries.

Human Eye Anatomy

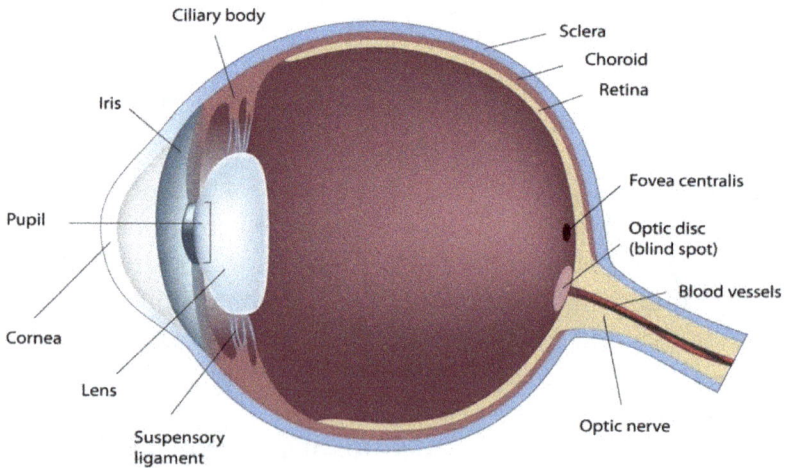

Alila Medical Media/Shutterstock.com

Protective structures for the eye include the orbital bone which surrounds the eye, eyelids, eyelashes, eyebrows, and the tears that come from the lacrimal glands with ducts that keep the eyes lubricated, moist, and clean. The sebaceous glands produce oil to keep the eyelids from sticking together.

The eyeball is fitted with muscles to support it and cause it to move to widen our field of vision. It has a vascular segment for circulation and the nerve portion called the optic nerve, located at the back of the eye. Damage to the optic nerve can cause partial or total blindness.

The numerous parts of the eye include the first layer, the sclera, the white part of the eye that gives it shape, stability, and protection. The optic nerve passes through the sclera at the back of the eye. The cornea is a transparent coat that covers the colored part of the eye and the pupil, which is the black hole in the middle of the iris where light enters the eyeball.

The second layer contains muscles, blood vessels, and the iris. The iris regulates the amount of light entering the eye by dilating or contracting to adjust for brightness or darkness of the viewing area. Another marvelous invention, design, and construction project here is the amazing system for altering the blood to make it clear in this area so that the blood cells do not interfere with the light coming in through the pupil.

Even the structure of the tissue here is changed from a rope type of assembly to an open weave. This also improves clarity for the light entering our eyes. How brilliant is that?

The third layer of the eye on the inside is the retina. Its primary function is to register images. God has built multiple neurons into our retinas which are called rods and cones. They can register all shades of color and images and then accurately emit the necessary electrical impulses to the occipital area of our brain for translation into visual images.

Another wonderful invention built into our sight system is the coordinated double image from our two separated eyes to give us depth perception, distance, and a more interesting three-dimensional imagery.

It is often claimed by evolutionists that the human retina is poorly designed because light must travel through nerves and blood vessels to reach the photoreceptor cells which are located *behind* the eye's wiring. However, there are many specific reasons for this placement of the photoreceptors.

A major one is that it allows close association between the rods and cones and the pigment epithelium system which is required to maintain the photoreceptors. It is also essential for the proper retinal functions. Both the rods and cones must physically interact with retinal pigment epithelial cells, which provide nutrients to the retina, recycles photo pigments, and creates an opaque layer to absorb excess light. [4]

The interior of the eye has an anterior and posterior chamber containing fluids and gels between which sits the transparent body called the lens. For vision to occur, light must pass through all of these structures. The lens and pupil accommodate refraction of the light waves to converge on the retina with the amount of light that allows us to see. The pupil narrows in bright sunlight and opens wider in the dark of night.

These are a few of the basic principles about sight which only hints at the complexity of the work that goes into the design and construction of our eyes for our marvelous vision. (Recall Darwin quote #3, Chapter 1, page 3). This is something that we can truly appreciate in our beautiful world.

2. Our Sense of Hearing

Isn't it great to be able to hear our favorite music, the nice words of our loved ones, the singing of birds, and the wind in the trees?

The ear is another organ that is amazingly made. Although we usually see only the outer ear called the pinna, we might not consider how the ear functions with all its intricacies involved. The ear has two important functions: (1) to register and transmit auditory sensations to our brain (hearing), and (2) to maintain our equilibrium (keep balance), both of which are critical to our lifestyle. Our ears are designed and built with devices that register sound waves and accurately transmit this information to our brains. Our ears are also built with brilliant parts which help us keep our balance.

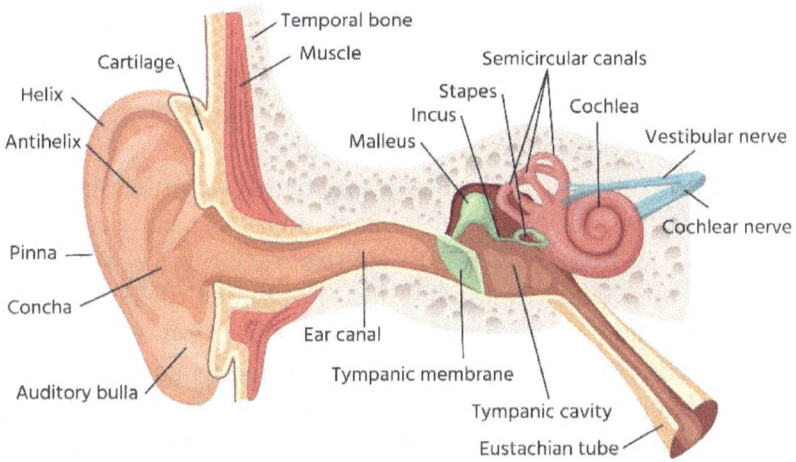

Tartila /Shutterstock

The ear consists of three sections: the outer (external), the middle, and the inner ear. All parts are vital and can be somewhat disabling if damaged.

The visible part of the ear is called the pinna. Attached to the head by muscles and ligaments, it is shaped specifically to pick up sounds of most meaning to humans, such as voices, warning sounds and music. It also protects the inner working mechanisms of the ear. From the pinna, an external canal leads into the eardrum. The highly sensitive skin inside the canal contains many mini-hairs and cerumen (ear wax) to prevent foreign bodies from entering the internal ear. At the end of this canal lies the eardrum or tympanic membrane, also covered with skin with a mucous membrane inside. Since this membrane is easily penetrated, great care must be taken not to push anything into the ear canal.

The middle ear is an air-filled cavity that communicates through the mastoid cells in the temporal bone and then into the auditory (Eustachian) tube leading to the throat. This serves to equalize pressure on both sides of the eardrum to prevent rupture. Three very tiny bones, the smallest in the body, called the malleus (hammer), incus (anvil), and stapes (stirrup) are connected by synovial (hinge) joints. They connect the eardrum to the inner ear and are attached to each other by ligaments.

59

The inner ear, called "the labyrinth," consists of cavities called vestibules, a cochlea (coiled hollow tube), and semi-circular canals. Fluid surrounds this area and all its parts which are connected by many sacs and canals. Tiny hairs, both inside and outside the cochlea, help transmit sound.

Basic ear physiology involves sound waves which are caught and directed by the pinna, then pass down the ear canal to the eardrum. Low-frequency sounds cause slow vibration, while high-frequency ones cause rapid vibration. The three little bones vibrate accordingly and pass the sound waves through the inner ear system to the cochlea. For hearing to result, inner ear mechanisms, pushing back and forth, stimulate the auditory nerve to carry sound signals to the correct part of our brain that translates sound to understanding.

Equilibrium is controlled by three semicircular canals located in the inner ear. They face in different directions to sense the three-dimensional world and contain many hairs of different lengths and consistencies. A gelatin-like fluid flows through and moves the hairs to stimulate sensory neurons that activate nerves to help maintain balance if your head position changes.

It requires a supernatural being to invent, design, and construct this marvelous hearing and balancing mechanism for each one of us.

3. Our Sense of Touch

With the amazing help of our approximately 100,000 miles of nerve "wiring", our brain can detect the exact point of a touch on our skin. Our sense of touch works when our skin comes in contact with different objects that register hot or cold, stillness, vibration, texture, tickling, tingling, pain, and pressure.

Our skin, the largest sense organ in our body, is composed of three layers. The epidermis is the outside layer, which we can see. It contains many sensitive cells that receive information about the environment that it touches. The next layer is the dermis which contains touch receptors that have more neurons in some areas than others, and hair follicles with nerve endings. More epidermal cells are formed here and rise to the top to replace dead epidermal cells which are sloughed off and help to create the dust that covers our tables. Oil and sweat glands are also part of the dermis layer. The third layer is a fatty pad that helps keep heat in our body and reduces damage to underlying structures. Intact skin also serves as a barrier to prevent germs from entering our body.

THE SKIN

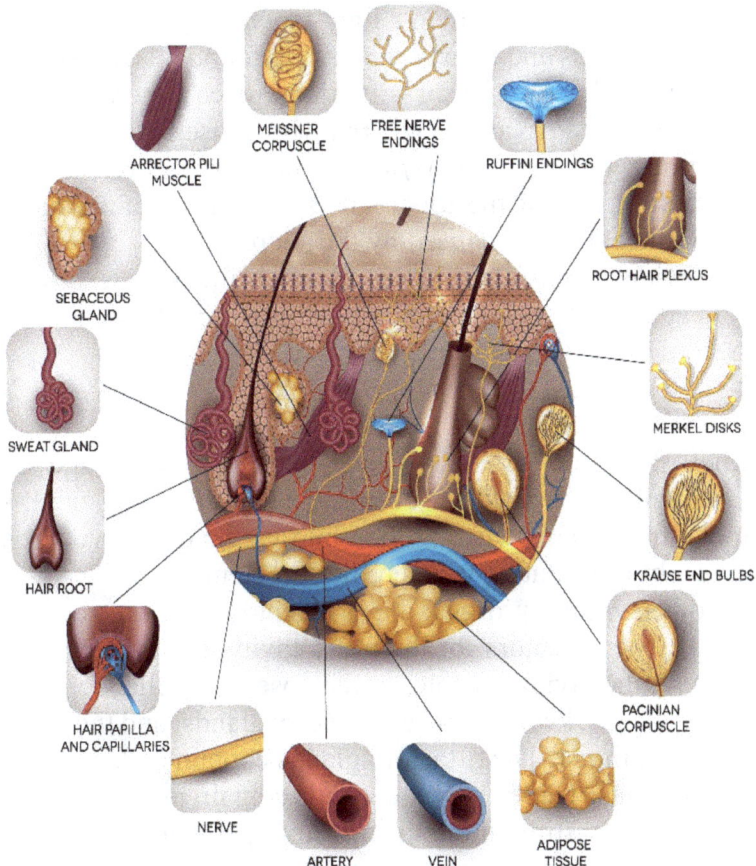

ARRECTOR PILI MUSCLE

MEISSNER CORPUSCLE

FREE NERVE ENDINGS

RUFFINI ENDINGS

SEBACEOUS GLAND

ROOT HAIR PLEXUS

SWEAT GLAND

MERKEL DISKS

HAIR ROOT

KRAUSE END BULBS

HAIR PAPILLA AND CAPILLARIES

PACINIAN CORPUSCLE

NERVE

ARTERY

VEIN

ADIPOSE TISSUE

Tefi/Shutterstock

The sense of touch is a greatly beneficial gift to us. By touching items we can determine size, shape, temperature, texture, and many other attributes. The sense of touch also relates us to our surrounding world, helping us walk, sit, and balance ourselves. For our safety we need many nerve endings and receptors to recognize hot, cold, and pain. This helps us to avoid burning, freezing, or otherwise damaging our flesh. Detecting vibrations and even a loving touch like a hug or a kiss are helpful and enjoyable. The desire for touch to show affection is very strong.

The brain can detect the exact point of touch. Our fingertips are particularly sensitive. When they are moved over an area, they can give details that no other skin area can. Pressure sensations on deeper tissues last longer than a light touch.

Pain sensations and their receptors are found all over our body. When hot, cold, pressure, or vibrations reach a certain level of intensity, pain can occur. Pain may be caused by burns, cuts, insect stings, bites, or a nervous system disfunction. Excessive stimulation of any of the touch areas can cause pain which can help minimize damage caused by the source.

It is evident that our skin senses are brilliantly designed and built, in addition to being carefully and precisely "wired" into our brain from every part of our body.

4. Our Sense of Smell

Smell does not just tell us of a good or bad change in our environment. Many critical events are identified by smell, such as smoke from a house fire or food burning on our stove. Loss of smell can be debilitating or even life-threatening.

All of our sensory organs have receptors that are required to function. The receptors for the nasal cavity are on either side of the septum, the dividing center of the nose. Epithelial cells, which produce mucous, keep the nose, olfactory glands, and the air going to our lungs, moist. The olfactory glands contain cells with helper bipolar neurons. The ends of these cells contain multiple hairs that react to odors by stimulating the olfactory pathway. This pathway leads to our brain's cerebral cortex where it is determined what odors are present. Thus, we smell. This entire process happens in about two seconds.

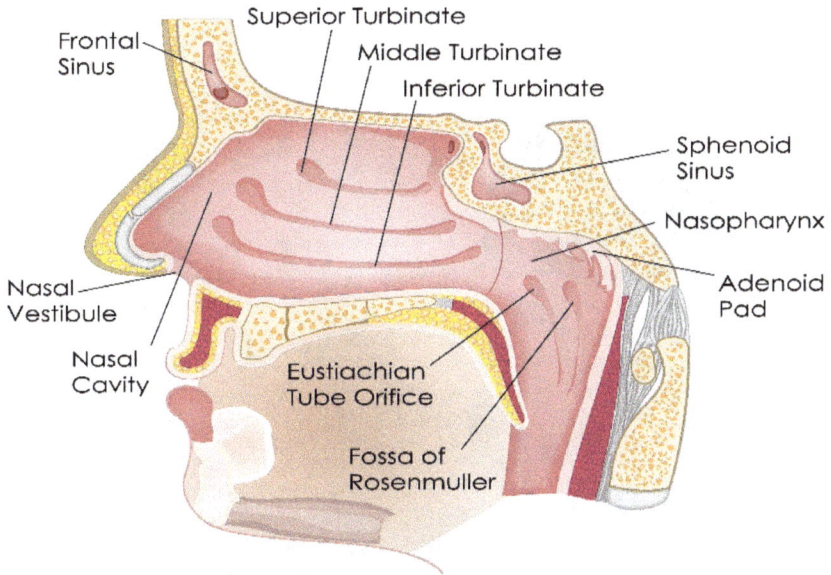

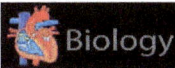

Biology **Nose Structure**

Snapgalleria/Shutterstock

Before we can smell a substance, it must enter into a gaseous, water-soluble state so that it can enter the nostrils sensory system and dissolve. Taking a deep breath and sniffing increases the smell acuity. The membranes of the olfactory hairs are mainly lipids (fats that are water-insoluble). To initiate the impulse to smell, the substance to be smelled must penetrate that lipid layer. Many different theories attempt to explain the complexity of how the nose smells. The most common is the small receptors are like a keyhole and the smell like a lock. If the two fit, the smell traits are registered; if not, no odor is sensed.

Any problems along this information route can cause disturbances with our sense of smell. Loss of smell can be a distressing experience.

As with our other senses, you can imagine the divine design and construction required to create a remarkable function like smelling.

5. Our Sense of Taste

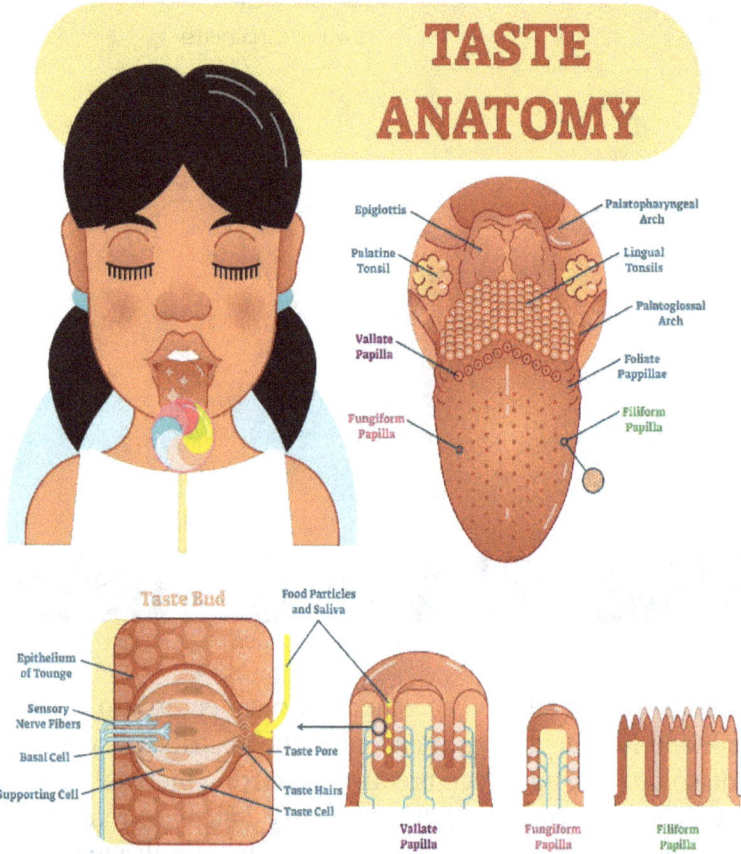

TASTE ANATOMY

Epiglottis

Palatine Tonsil

Vallate Papilla

Fungiform Papilla

Palatopharyngeal Arch

Lingual Tonsils

Palatoglossal Arch

Foliate Pappillae

Filiform Papilla

Taste Bud

Food Particles and Saliva

Epithelium of Tounge

Sensory Nerve Fibers

Basal Cell

Supporting Cell

Taste Pore

Taste Hairs

Taste Cell

Vallate Papilla

Fungiform Papilla

Filiform Papilla

Vector Mine/Shutterstock

The receptors for our taste – also called gustatory sensations – are located in our taste buds. Each taste bud contains multiple taste cells that allow us to recognize the flavors of sweet, salt, sour, bitter, and savory. Each taste bud is "wired" to register and transmit the information to the correct part of our brain.

The taste buds are located under the mucous membrane of the tongue in the rough, wart-like surfaces called papillae. Of various shapes and sizes, these papillae are able to identify the five tastes.

The large papillae at the base of the tongue contain thousands of taste buds. On the tongue's upper surface are thousands of other smaller papillae. Each taste bud identifies different levels of intensity.

As with other body cells, the taste buds are replaced once a week. These papillae contain a small opening connected to a saliva gland which provides this initial digestive solution to what we eat. Saliva also helps sensitize our taste buds, thereby increasing our ability to appreciate the taste of our food. From there, nerve cells identify the substances we have ingested. After contact with the food, the taste receptors react rapidly. Smell is also brought into play to help the taste buds determine the traits of the substance tasted. The combination of odors and taste involves a psychological adaptation in the brain so that specific tastes can rapidly be determined and differentiated.

The front of the tongue recognizes sweeter tastes, the sides of the tongue detect salt, savory, and sour flavors, and the back picks up bitter tastes. Since all people are different, the intensity and pleasure or displeasure of each taste is individualistic.

With this quick look at all five of our senses, isn't it truly amazing how marvelously our Creator has made each one of us?

Applications for Life:

1. About how many correct atoms per second have to be found, selected, counted, and precisely assembled to build the replacement red blood cells for a 150 lb. male? _____

2. Where do all these atoms come from? _____

_____

3. Why is it important to eat good food and breathe good air?

_____

_____

4. About how many miles of nerve fibers have to be constructed and maintained just for our brain? _____

5. What has to be added to new cells to give life and function to the inanimate atoms used to construct the cell?

_____

6. The design sketch for the superintelligent and careful work for constructing our eyes is shown on page 56. What other features does our Creator build to protect our phenomenal eyes?

_____

_____

_____

7. Do you think that highly complex sensory organs like our ears could be built of atoms by an unintelligent process, or yourself, or even a great scientist? Why or why not? _____

_____

_____

8. Looking at the diagram of our skin, how much intelligence and care do you think it takes to build this covering for our body?

_____

_____

9. Another highly complex organ that is very beneficial to us is our nose. List five types of things you can smell that you like, or are important to you. _____

_____

10.   List five types of things you like to taste or are important for you to taste. _____

_____

_____

References and Notes:

[1] Regarding the enormous work performed for each of us just in constantly replacing our red blood cells:

Pallister, C.J., *Haematology: Biomedical Science Explained,* Butterworth-Heinemann, Burlington, MA, 1999. He states that an average 70 kg adult male produces about 2,300,000 red blood cells every second.
Tortora, G. J., *Principles of Anatomy and Physiology,* John Wiley & Sons, New York, NY, 2008. He states that there are approximately 280,000,000 molecules of hemoglobin per red blood cell.
Perutz, Max, *Science Is Not A Quiet Life: Unraveling the Atomic Mechanism of Haemoglobin,* World Scientific Publishing Company, Hackensack, NJ, 1997. He states that each hemoglobin molecule contains approximately 10,000 atoms.

[2]   Wedeen, Van, and L.L. Wald, in article "Secrets of the Brain" by Carl Zimmer, *National Geographic,* February, 2014, p. 34.

[3]   Ham, K., P. Varnum, and D. Mason, (Producers), P. Varnum, (Director), *Fearfully and Wonderfully Made,* DVD, Answers in Genesis Productions, Hebron, KY, 2007.

[4] Bergman, Jerry. *The "Poor Design" Argument Against Intelligent Design Falsified*, Bartlett Publishing, Tulsa, OK, 2019.

Chapter 5
Our Incredible Molecular Machines

What Are the Molecular Machines Within Our Cells?

The more we learn about the amazing variety of phenomenal works carried on within our cells, the more we realize that cells cannot be constructed without an omniscient designer and builder. The James Tour Group at Rice University has developed a number of relatively simple molecular machines, as have the 2016 Nobel Prize winners for Chemistry, Sauvage, Stoddart, and Feringa, as well as other groups working on similar projects.

"The first step towards a molecular machine was taken by Jean-Pierre Sauvage in 1983, when he succeeded in linking two ring-shaped molecules together to form a chain, called a catenane. Fraser Stoddart took the second step in 1991, when he developed rotaxane. He threaded a molecular ring onto a thin molecular axle and demonstrated that the ring was able to move along the axle. Bernard Feringa was the first person to develop a molecular motor; in 1999 he got a molecular rotor blade to spin continually in the same direction." [1]

The James Tour Group invested over a decade of expensive research and development to produce their first simplistic molecular machine made of just one single molecule. It can actually move with the help of stimuli such as ultraviolet light. The assembly and testing of some of these sub-microscopic units must be performed on a flat gold surface heated to between 170°C and 225°C (338°F - 437°F). [2]

The many, almost infinitely more complex molecular machines constructed within most of our cells are created at body temperature (37°C = 98.6°F) without the need for ultraviolet light, flat gold surfaces, large, specialized equipment, high-powered microscopes, etc. plus unworkable lengths of time.

Far more intelligence is essential for our cell construction than scientists can achieve at this time. We can build only extremely simple units by comparison to our Creator's handiwork. We also cannot build any significant single part of a cell from raw materials, and we cannot provide the "breath of life" to anything.

This is why we have included in Chapter 7, one of the principles of life under "Dead Dogs Don't Bark." "Although the dog has every needed atom and molecule precisely assembled and placed for its eyes, ears, nose, teeth, heart, legs, brain, etc., without the "'breath of life,'" it is not going to move itself one millimeter."

So why would anyone think that something with no intelligence, like evolution, could do all this superintelligent life-causing work?

The theory of evolution as the cause of life is now considered by many to be *"factually falsified," and that is a very good thing for our nations.*

It is time for science teachers to teach truth and "go where the evidence leads, without reprisal," especially in the field of constructing living cells and entities, including us.

Many of the molecular machines in our cells are irreducibly complex, meaning they could not function without having all their parts in place, including the "breath of life", from their beginning. This is another strike against the theory of (slow change) evolution as the cause of life.

Consider Darwin's theory of origins whereby there was (theoretically) a common ancestor for all species at the base of his "tree of life". The theory surmises that an original cell was spontaneously created in some speculative primordial pond. This cell would have needed the ability to find and process nourishment for its survival, to reproduce itself, to pass on its best traits and make many improvements to its design over many generations, eventually becoming fish, birds, mammals, primates, and people. Darwin was unsure how this could happen but assumed that it did and produced his theory from this supposition.

Many things were unknown about atoms, molecules, cells, and life at the time Darwin published his first book on evolution in 1859. Although he admitted that there were a number of ways his theory could "absolutely break down," he ignored them or tried to rationalize them away.

After long study, many evolutionists, as well as former evolutionists, agree that the original reproducing cell could never have appeared by chance no matter how much time was available. We are now learning more about the phenomenal complexities essential for the many different molecular machines that are assembled in most of our cells to enable them to function.

All of these various phenomenal little machines have to be constructed within our cells, using the correct numbers of the right types of atoms, all precisely assembled and fastened together in proper sequence, and with the "breath of life" added to make them live and function.

The communication system within each cell must be intelligently constructed and guided to help with each cell's proper assembly and functioning. For example, at each cell-construction site, choices and decisions have to be made as to: what nutrient atoms are required to be extracted from the adjacent blood vessels; where these nutrients need to be placed; how to deliver them to that place; what parts of the cell need repairing or replacing; when and how to do each particular task; and when the entire cell needs replacing.

A full description of all the types of molecular machines and their sub-varieties in our cells would require a large book, but a few examples are:

Kinesin, which is a marvelous little workhorse designed and constructed within most of our cells, to transport various cargo loads from one area of its cell to another, both where and when needed. It literally has two 'feet' to walk along a tube concurrently built ahead of it from where it has to fetch a particular cargo to transport this cargo to where it is needed. It has two little 'hands' to hold the cargo as it flips one foot in front of the other along each newly tube-road which is, after use, removed so the cell does not get cluttered. The animated online videos of these amazing live machines shows them doing their jobs. [4]

Myosin, can also deliver cargo in our cells, and a variant of myosin helps our muscles to contract by converting chemical energy to physical energy for that purpose.

Proteasome is a large group of proteins that act as waste disposer machines. When cell proteins are damaged or worn out, they are tagged, unfolded, and cut into small pieces called peptides. Then the proteasome disposes of them through a cell portal and into the bloodstream to be delivered to our waste system.

A lysosome is similar to a proteasome, but it breaks up an entire cell part or whole cell that is then delivered to our waste system.

A calcium pump is the molecular machine that pumps calcium ions across our cell membranes using a four-step process.

Ribosomes are particles God makes to convert the RNA instructional code in our cells to manufacture various proteins. The mRNA is originally copied from the instruction code in our DNA.

A mitochondrion contains many enzymes which help to convert the food nutrients delivered to our cells, into usable energy. It does this by charging ADP (adenosine diphosphate) like a battery is charged by electricity. When charged, it is ATP (adenosine triphosphate), an energy-storage and energy-carrying molecule.

ATP Synthase is a complex molecular machine with a mass equivalent to that of about 500,000 hydrogen atoms. It is hyper-intelligently constructed to operate at about 6000 rpm within the mitochondria membrane. Its function is to generate energy for physiological reactions like muscle contraction.

The Nucleolus, often called the "brain" of the cell, takes up around 25% of the volume of the nucleus. It is constructed of proteins and ribonucleic acids (RNA). Its functions include processing ribosomal RNA (rRNA) and combining it with proteins to produce functional ribosomes.

Casey Luskin of the Discovery Institute has compiled a list of 40 of the different types of molecular machines constructed for our life.[5]

The more we learn about our amazing 'Life,' the more fascinating and gratifying is the wondrous care provided for us. We just have to select healthful foods and healthful habits so that our Creator can help us have our best well-being.

Applications for Life

1.   Which two groups of scientists are credited here for proving mankind does not have the intelligence and skills required to construct the complex molecular machines for our bodies?

_____

_____

2.   About how many years did it take the 2016 Nobel Prize winners in Chemistry to develop their relatively simple molecular machines and receive their Prize? _____

3.   What type of surface was required for building the molecular machines and what temperature range?

_____

4. In the degree of complexity, how do these man-made molecular machines compare to those made by our Creator for our cells?

_____

5.   What significant factors do the molecular machines made for our cells have that the man-made ones do not have?

_____

_____

6.   What type of action has been proven essential for the construction of living molecular machines for our cells?

_____

7.   Does the process of evolution have the intelligence required to construct the many molecular machines needed for our cells?

_____

References and Notes:

[1] Sauvage, J-P., J.F. Stoddart, and B.L. Feringa, http://www.nobelprize.org/nobel-prizes/chemistry/laureates/2016/press.html http://www.nobelprize.org/nobel-prizes/chemistry/laureates/2016/press.htmlprizes/chemistry/laureates/2016/press.html ,- accessed November 28, 2016.

[2] Tour, James, www.jmtour.com/about/research: http://www.jmtour.com/about/research-information accessed November 28, 2016.

[3] Meyer, Stephen C., *Signature in the Cell,* Harper Collins, New York, NY, 2009, p. 201.

[4] See YouTube, "The Workhorse of the Cell: Kinesin" by Discovery Science News.

[5] Luskin, Casey, *Molecular Machines in the Cell,* Discovery Institute, 2010, www.discovery.org/a/14791 , accessed November 28, 2016

Chapter 6
Is Atomic Biology Falsifiable?

What is incorrect about this newly discovered science?

THE BASIC PREMISES OF ATOMIC BIOLOGY:

- All living cells are constructed using atoms as building blocks;

- Atoms have no intelligence or internal means to move themselves into their precise location in a designated cell part, therefore they require an intelligent external being to place them properly;

- Cell parts are made of specific numbers of specific atoms precisely assembled in the proper sequence and position in order for life to occur;

- Specific complex molecular machines must be precisely constructed for specific types of cells;

- It has been (unintentionally) shown by the 2016 Nobel Prize winners in Chemistry (Sauvage, Stoddart, and Feringa) and many other scientists that humans have nowhere near enough intelligence, skills, or tools to construct even the simplest living molecular machines using raw elements. Thus, a "superintelligent" cause (having far more intelligence than humans) is essential for building cell parts, cells, and living entities;

- There is only one such superintelligent being known to mankind that can, and has, achieved this goal, and that is the entity known by our governments and the majority of our citizens as our Creator, God.

- As evolution, by definition, has no intelligence to use, it is incapable and thus factually falsified as being both the origin and the cause of life.

This book contains many proofs for the essentiality of intelligent work for building cells, including a four-step scientific method discussed in the following chapter. Any one of these proofs is sufficient to falsify Darwinism as the best explanation for the cause of life.

Many hypotheses exist endeavoring to explain how living entities are constructed without the need for a superintelligent mind. However, each one has unbridgeable gaps and falls short of adequacy.

All that is required to falsify "atomic biology" as the correct explanation for the cause of life, is to show that no intelligent physical work is required to find, sort, select, count, and precisely assemble, all the exact numbers of the correct atoms to construct each living cell part and cell required for life.

To simplify the challenge even further, just prove that the atoms for constructing the four DNA bases, adenine ($C_5H_5N_5$), guanine ($C_5H_5N_5O_1$), cytosine ($C_4H_5N_3O_1$), and thymine ($C_5H_6N_2O_2$) do not require to be intelligently selected from an adjacent source, nor do the atoms need to be intelligently and carefully counted, nor do these atoms have to be precisely assembled. These achievements will falsify "atomic biology" as the best explanation of the true cause of life.

Clearly, the precisely counted numbers of the correct element atoms must be carefully selected from an available source and carefully assembled. Each step requires intelligent action, and evolution, by definition, is void of intelligence.

The essentiality of superintelligent physical works with atoms for constructing living cell parts, cells, and entities is a "show-stopper" for evolution as the true origin and cause of life.

Education leaders will lose their credibility and respect *if* they continue to enforce the teaching of false information regarding the cause of life and *disallow* the teaching of evidence-based science wherever it leads.

Applications for Life:

1. The building blocks for constructing cell parts, cells, and us, are

    _____

2. Why can't atoms move themselves into their proper place in a cell part?

    _____

    _____

3. Would any random types or numbers of atoms work for building a molecular machine for a cell? Why or why not?

    _____

    _____

4. Why do different types of molecular machines have to be constructed for different types of cells?

    _____

    _____

    _____

5. How do we know that scientists do not have the required skills to build the molecular machines for our cells?

    _____

    _____

6. What entity or being does have enough intelligence and care to build our cell parts and cells for us?

_____

7. What would it take to show that our Creator is not the cause of our life?

_____

_____

_____

_____

Chapter 7
Moving Darwinism, Neo-Darwinism, and Macroevolution to the History Department

A MAJOR PROBLEM FOR WESTERN SOCIETY

Madelyn Murray O'Hair and friends were only one group whose work began to destroy Western society from within. The atheistic religion of Humanism expressed in their magazine, *The Humanist,* (January-February, 1983), this clarion call: *"The battle for mankind's future must be waged and won in the public-school classroom by teachers who correctly perceive their roles as the proselytizers of a new faith.... these teachers must embody the same selfless dedication as the most rabid fundamentalist preachers, for they will be ministers of another sort, utilizing the classroom instead of the pulpit to convey humanist values in whatever subject they teach, regardless of educational level - pre-school, day-care or large state university. The classroom must and will become an arena of conflict between the old and the new - the rotting corpse of Christianity, together with all its adjacent evils and misery, and the new faith of humanism."*

See also page 88 for more examples of organizations focusing on destroying our society. The Southern Poverty Law organization lists hundreds of "Hate and Anti-Governemnt" organizations.

To counter this severe attack, through the last 32 years, with help from 20 PhD.s, 9 DScs, 3 MDs, 3 Mathematicians, 2 MScs, and 8 Independent Researchers, we have significantly added to the existing strong evidence for falsifying the destructive Theory of Evolution as both the origin and the cause of life. We have also made the case for the essentiality of a superintelligent being to construct every living cell part, cell, and entity.

Through this work, we have developed a new, more logical, and accurate science to replace all Darwinisms as the taught cause of life in our educational systems, i.e. "Atomic Biology."

We believe that mainstream science has avoided focusing on the atomic assembly level in biological cell construction because enormous numbers of decisions, choices, atom selections, counting, and precision assembly work must be performed at this level. This requires superintelligent work with atoms, and evolutionism is devoid of intelligence.

Thousands of scientists have openly declared their skepticism of evolution as the cause of life, and God only knows how many other scientists, teachers, professors, and medical professionals there are who dare not make their skepticism known for fear of losing their tenure, careers, or earned reputation. ***This enforced restriction is absolutely anti-science and must be outlawed. It is holding back scientific progress and misleading students.***

To provide clarity, we first require specific definitions of the terms "Darwinism," "Neo-Darwinism," and "macroevolution" that we are dealing with in this project. These terms are not to be confused with "microevolution" which is not evolution per se but simply minor changes in details like hair color, skin color, eye color, or size. There are definite boundaries to the types of changes controlled by our Creator.

The "evolution" we are referring to is that taught in our public schools, colleges, and universities. The three similar forms of evolution, "Darwinism," "Neo-Darwinism," and "macroevolution," are all attempts to explain the origin and cause of life whereby all species and kinds had a "common ancestor."

These visions of evolution surmise that this first organism was constructed by an unguided, random event billions of years ago. "Natural selection" is included as one aspect of evolution as an extension of "*survival*-of-the-fittest" plants and animals, but it does not explain the "*arrival* (origin) of the fittest."

Evolution teaching is that these changes happened by random mutations that provided improvements in ascending offspring. There was no guidance, purpose, design or intelligence involved in this theoretical process. No God or intelligence is allowed to be taught in the construction of living entities.

It is now widely understood that no random process could produce even the simplest reproducing cell with its essential highly complex functioning systems. It would need the complex molecular machines for its functions of obtaining nourishment, digesting that, and reproducing itself with improvements. The offspring would have needed these complex capabilities produced quickly and accurately enough for the entity to survive.

A key fact is that even our top scientists do not have anywhere near enough ability to build the simplest of living molecular machines using atoms, let alone an entire living cell. We cannot generate life from non-living atoms today, even with our vast scientific knowledge and highly sophisticated equipment.

As Sir Fred Hoyle and his long-term associate, Chandra Wickramasinghe, who were Cambridge University astronomers and physicists stated, *"The likelihood of the formation of life from inanimate matter* [without intelligent help] *is one to a number with 40,000 noughts* [zeroes] *after it. . . . It is big enough to bury Darwin and the whole theory of evolution."* [1]

Dr. Stephen C. Meyer, an advocate of intelligent design and cofounder of the Discovery Institute's Center for Science and Culture, stated in his book, *Signature in the Cell, "The* simplest *extant* (still surviving) *cell,* Mycoplasma genitalium – *a tiny bacterium that inhabits the human urinary tract – requires 'only' 482 proteins to perform its necessary functions and 562,000 bases of DNA (just under 1,200 base pairs per gene) ... .*

Based upon minimal-complexity experiments, some scientists speculate (but have not demonstrated) that a simple one-cell organism might have been able to survive with as few as 250 to 400 genes." [2]

Now, the teaching of Darwinisms as the origin and cause of life should be banned by the Supreme Court of the USA.

The problem of mutations as the creator

Darwinism theorizes an explanation for the progression from molecules to cells, to bacteria-like life forms, to amphibians, reptiles, mammals, primates, and, lastly, to humans purely by the accumulation of **mutations** that produce the genetic variety required to evolve new life forms. This genetic variety, evolution-ists argue, is selected by natural selection, a process called "surviv-al of the fittest" whereby some animals that are more fit, are more likely to survive than others. These would improve the species, and, the theory postulates, cause evolution into new species.

In short, modern Darwinism teaches that we, and all life, are the product of billions of damage events to the genome called genetic mutations, which due to survival-of-the-fittest law, make fitter life-forms that are more likely to survive. Far more mutations are destructive than those that are productive in any living entity. These genetic damage events are caused by carcinogens, including dangerous radiation such as gamma and cosmic rays, and mutagenic chemicals, such as tobacco smoke.

It is difficult to know what percentage of scientists actually believe the view that mutations and natural selection are our creator, not God. Penalties are severe for scientists, especially teachers and professors, who openly mention that they believe in God, or even intelligence as the Creator.

This restriction is *anti-science* of the worst kind.

The exact percentages of those who believe in God vs. those who believe in evolution as the cause of life, are unknowable at this time but we do have some estimates. See Bob Enyart's research on page 261.

The recent discoveries of the phenomenal complexities in molecular machinery constructed within cells, have changed the minds of former evolutionists brave enough to admit their skepticism regarding evolution as the builder, sustainer, and maintainer of all living cells and entities.

Supporters of the idea that humans, and all creatures, are the result of billions of genetic mutations, have a view that is radically contrary to observable facts. This erroneous theory of evolution must be taught in public schools as fact, whether believed or not, mainly because the lower courts have ruled it so. Furthermore, information contrary to this view must not be taught because the courts have ruled that doing so is teaching back-door religion (misinterpreted separation of church and state clause) and is thusly, unconstitutional in the U.S.A. This is an enormous mistake because *the Creator who is the God of our government, is **not** "the church". The church cannot create any living entity.*

Because only evolution as the cause of life has been allowed to be taught in our public schools since the 1960s, and because secular scientists have controlled most of the media regarding science book and journal publishing, most people in the Western world, even many people who call themselves Christians, have been influenced to accept Darwinisms as true. *However, accumulating discoveries showing the phenomenal complexities in the construction, sustenance, maintenance and operation of cell parts, now shows even evolutionists that mankind does not have the knowledge, intelligence, or ability to do this work. Therefore, **evolution, having no intelligence, is now factually falsified as both the origin and the cause of life,** and this is a very good factor for our nations.* It just has to be publicized.

As the theory of evolution is now factually falsified as an accurate explanation of the origin and cause of life, it should be moved to the history department and replaced with a more accurate and truthful life science.

Using the proper chemical elements and the greatest related scientific intelligence and sophisticated equipment available today, our scientists cannot assemble even <u>one</u> live, functioning organelle or molecular machine, such as a mitochondrion or a kinesin, using raw elements, e.g. making a carrot cell out of dirt.

Knowing these facts, can anyone seriously believe that anything as complex as an entire cell could be assembled into living existence without an intelligent creator?

Our objective is to provide solid evidence for scientific determination that the 'theory of evolution' is now *factually falsified* regarding the origin and cause of life. It should be disqualified from education curricula and moved to the 'History-of-failed-theories' Department. This suggested action is based on the belief that the majority of teachers and professors would prefer a legacy of following evidence and teaching truth as opposed to teaching verified fallacy.

In science, a hypothesis or theory must be testable to evaluate it for falsifiability. The concept that God's creative work cannot be evaluated for falsifiability is false.

God's role as creator, sustainer, maintainer, repairer, and provider of the "breath of life" to our otherwise inanimate atoms, is falsifiable. We just have to show how all of the physical work of finding the right numbers of the right atoms in soil, air, and water, as well as the sorting, selecting, counting, grasping, precisely placing, and fastening them in their correct position in each cell of our foods, and then the redoing of all these brilliant works with these atoms at lightning speed to build our various cell parts and cells, with all the decisions and choices this requires, can be performed with no intelligent guidance whatsoever.

Considering that with the intelligence and scientific knowledge mankind has accumulated, and the sophisticated equipment we have devised, and that this is totally insufficient to construct even one of the simplest molecular machines for one living cell, it is obvious that far greater intelligence than ours is essential for creating life.

Until it can be shown that this enormous amount of supreme-minded decision-making and physical work with atoms can be performed without any intelligence or guidance, then Darwinism, Neo-Darwinism, and macroevolution should be set aside as unworkable, falsified, and obsolete theories for the cause of life.

These Darwinisms Do Not Stand Up to the Tests of Reason.

It is time for a replacement science and we believe that "Atomic Biology" deserves serious scholarly and truthful consideration.

Charles Darwin himself stated: *"If it could be demonstrated that any complex organ existed which could not possibly have been formed by numerous, successive slight modifications, my theory would absolutely break down."* [3]

Here is the demonstration:

In recent scientific developments, scientists Jean-Pierre Sauvage, Sir J. Fraser Stoddard, Bernard L. Feringa, and the James Tour Group, have shown how great the difficulty is in building and operating even the simplest of molecular machines. Their molecular machines are simplistic compared to any one of the

40 molecular machines built to operate within our cells. Many superintelligent decisions, choices, and physical works with atoms are essential for the construction of the complex cell machinery and organs of every living creature; evolution simply cannot perform these intelligent works because, by definition, it has no intelligence with which to do the work.

Darwin gave us several other reasons that would show how his theory of evolution could *"absolutely break down."* He knew these potential concerns even before today's knowledge of the complexity of life existed. For example, regarding the complexity of the eye, Darwin states: *"To suppose that the eye with all its inimitable contrivances for adjusting the focus to different distances, for admitting different amounts of light, and for the correction of spherical and chromatic aberration, could have been formed by natural selection, seems, I freely confess, absurd in the highest degree."* [4]

He continued however, supposing that from the most primitive light-sensing organ through heredity with modification, the eye could be initiated and improved to become its current status as an "organ of perfection and complication." Yet, since evolution and natural selection have no intelligence or mechanism to build even one eye cell, or any other cell from atoms, his theory, in reality, has "absolutely broken down."

Human Eye Anatomy

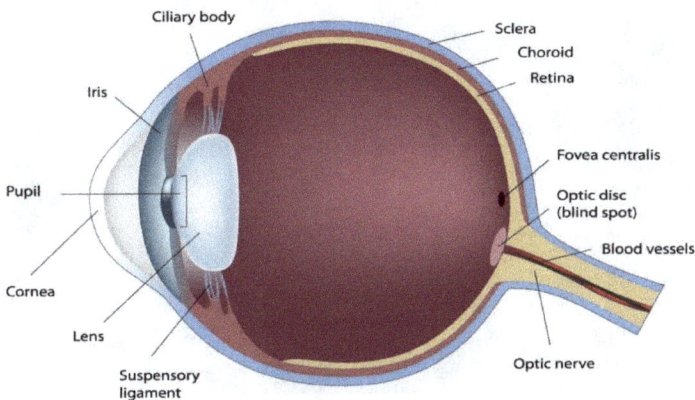

Alila Medical Media/Shutterstock.com

Without today's technology, Darwin could not have known exactly how phenomenally complex eyes are, nor did he understand the ultra-intelligent atomic works and care necessary for the construction, sustenance, maintenance, and repair of every cell involved in our eyesight.

In *Origins,* Darwin says of eyesight: *"[M]ay we not believe that a living optical instrument might thus be formed as superior to one of glass, as the Works of the Creator are* (superior) *to those of man."* [5] (Emphasis added).

Obviously, at the time of writing this in *Origins,* Darwin had great respect for the Creator and His superiority above man's abilities.

Regarding peacock's feathers, Darwin states, *"The sight of a feather in a peacock's tail, whenever I gaze at it, makes me feel sick!"* [6] It seems that the beauty of the design and construction of even one feather in a peacock's tail overwhelmed him....and his short-sighted explanation for it through his theory.

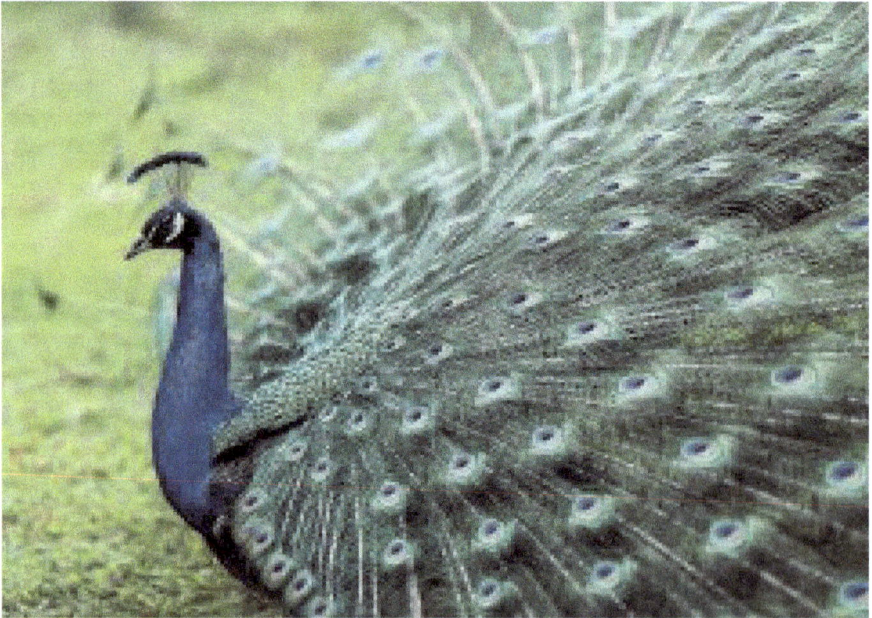

rickyd/shutterstock.com

If we consider the enormous, brilliant, caring work that goes into designing, constructing, sustaining, and maintaining a peacock's tail feather using atoms from the "dust," it should overwhelm us all.

This example of beauty in creatures must be primarily for God's own enjoyment and ours.

Darwin could not have known the details of the work involved in building living entities because the knowledge of the biological construction of cells using atoms was not available to him at that time.

Remember, atoms have no *internal* means to move themselves into a precise position in a cell, therefore, an *external* cause is required.

The current restrictions against teaching even the possibility of omniscient involvement in life do not change the reality that superintelligence, vision, dexterity, precision, care, and speed are essential for the life of each living entity.

Ignoring these facts does not change these facts. It is anti-science that should be outlawed. We are more than foolish to continue teaching the false information that is called Darwinism, Neo-Darwinism, and other macroevolutionary philosophies. We cripple our students, future scientists, and leaders by teaching false information.

It is more than just ridiculous to teach students to <u>pretend</u> that the intelligently designed features they observe in living plants and creatures are not intelligently designed and constructed..

It is important to remember that even with all of mankind's accumulated knowledge, specially developed equipment and chemical combinations, our scientists have not been able to come anywhere close to producing even one significant living part of any organism from unliving elements.

Is it not ironic to consider the huge amount of time, intelligence, effort, science, and money invested to prove that no intelligence is required to create a living cell? What this does prove is the exact opposite, that Superintelligence IS required. As scientists have learned more about the mind-boggling complexity of even the simplest cells, many are distancing themselves, both formally and informally, from belief in evolutionary dogma.

One brave group of scientists have signed a document titled "A Scientific Dissent from Darwinism".[7] There was no compulsion or duress placed on the scientists to sign the document. The term "brave" is used because many scientists, teachers, and public education institutes (perhaps the majority) are forced or intimidated into teaching only "macroevolution" or "Neo-Darwinism" as the cause of life, by *fear* of termination, penalty, lawsuit, or other despicable tactic – this is totally *anti-science.*

One movie documenting this disgraceful treatment of several scientists is titled, *"Expelled, No Intelligence Allowed"*. [8]

There are examples of other instances including this recent one: A college in Texas was recently intimidated into dropping a non-credit, night-school course on the controversy between Evolution and Intelligent Design. Ironically, the names of the intimidating groups portrayed freedom and free thinking in science with input from other science, and they had support from a 'liberty' organization.[9]

Their actions in this case went in the absolute opposite direction to the message in their names, i.e., antifreedom, anti-free thinking, anti-liberty, and anti-science, as science is supposed to go where the evidence leads.[10]

Another "liberty" organization is sometimes just as misleading and takes their victims, including public education institutions, to court to frustrate the *liberty* to teach in classrooms that there might be some intelligence in the way living entities are designed.

It appears that these organizations are using the 'liberty' of 'free thought' and broad 'freedoms' allowed by constitutional law, to destroy the 'liberty' of 'free thought' and certain 'freedoms' in our educational system.

How have we, in our democracies, allowed ourselves to be dictated into this abominable position in our education systems?

It goes against the beliefs and rights of the majority. ***Democracy is gone if a minority is allowed to rule unchecked, especially with our youth.***

*Good science is to be encouraged to go wherever the evidence leads. Science is supposed to be the search for truth. Any actions preventing that are **anti-science.***

Let's Clarify the Problem as Much as We Can

The unscientific shortcomings of the evolutionary doctrine exclusively taught in our secular education institutions, was summed up by an open and honest evolutionist, Harvard Professor Richard Lewontin. His words were, *"We take the side of (materialist) science in spite of the patent absurdity of some of its constructs, in spite of its failure to fulfill many of its extravagant promises of health and life, in spite of the tolerance of the scientific community for unsubstantiated just-so stories, because we have a prior commitment, a commitment to materialism. It is not that the methods and institutions of science somehow compel us to accept a material explanation of the phenomenal world, but, on the contrary, that we are forced by our a priori adherence to material causes to create an apparatus of investigation and a set of concepts that produce material explanations, no matter how counter-intuitive, no matter how mystifying to the uninitiated. Moreover, that materialism is absolute, **for we cannot allow a Divine Foot in the door.***" [11] (Emphasis added). **This is blatant anti-science.**

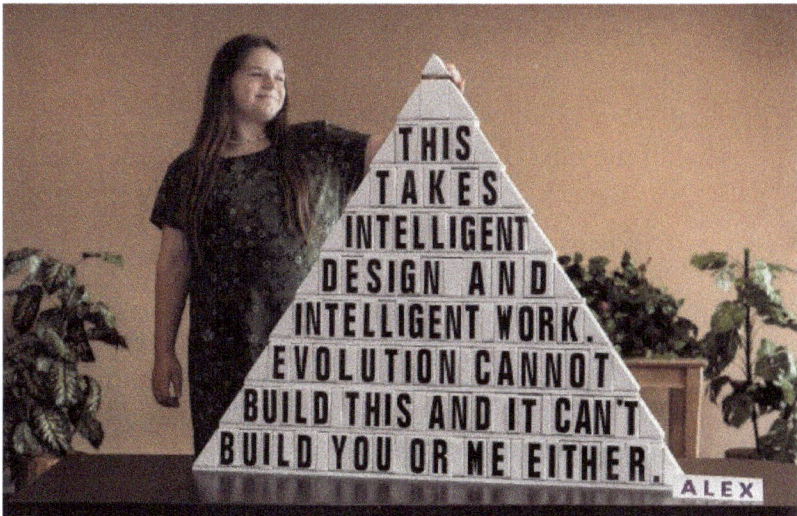

isphotography.com/realityrandd.com

That is right, Alex. "Evolution" (Darwinism/Macroevolution) cannot build anything because it does not have the required intelligence and other necessary capabilities.

By definition, evolution has no intelligence. So, how could "evolution" manufacture the right numbers of the right-sized building blocks, paint them, letter them, then grasp onto each one and precisely place it to build even this relatively simple, but significant, pyramid message?

Making these wooden building blocks did take some intelligent design and work, but it was extremely simple in comparison to the design and physical work involved in building each one of our trillions of living cells.

In an attempt to understand where the prompting for the anti-Creator thoughts are coming from, Chapter 8 will provide some further clues.

For good reasons, the four nations highlighted is this book were founded on Godly principles. According to census after census, the majority of the citizens in these countries continue to believe in Him. Some of the reasons they believe in God include their appreciation for the following:

- for the food that He makes for everyone (whether we thank Him or not);
- for healing our wounds;
- for answered prayers;
- for His guidance and wisdom;
- for the family and friends that God has made for us;
- for the beauty in the flowers, trees, pets, birds, and other creatures made for our enjoyment.

The majority of citizens do not have enough faith to believe atheism that teaches some random, unintelligent, accidental, unguided, or magical process created us and the universe.

Here are the words to a song named "Goodbye, Evolution,"sung by "Karen and the Kids":

"Satan uses Darwin's theory to make folks forget God,
But he can't fool all the people all the time.
God still faithfully makes our food from dust and rain,

And He makes our cells from our food; it's all Divine.
Evolution is the worst hoax of all time!
Oh, everything's made of atoms, and atoms don't have legs.
Mr. Darwin did not know this, but atoms don't have legs.
So, someone has to place each atom to build each living thing.
Atoms cannot jump to their right place; someone creates live things.
It really is so simple; the scientists could agree,
That everything's made of atoms, and atoms cannot see.
So, someone has to place each atom to build each living thing.
Atoms cannot jump to their right place; someone creates live things.
It has to be someone real smart 'cause I'm no piece of junk.
My trillions of cells each play their part; my builder is no punk.
Yes, someone has to place each atom to build each living thing.
Atoms cannot jump to their right place; someone creates live things.
So, goodbye evolution; to most you make no sense;
Except to population who haven't seen love immense.
But no one ever loves them more nor works so hard for them,
Than God their great Creator; all life depends on Him!
All life depends on Him! On Him! GOODBYE EVOLUTION !" [12]
     (available from iTunes)

Where Do Our Building-Block Atoms Come From?

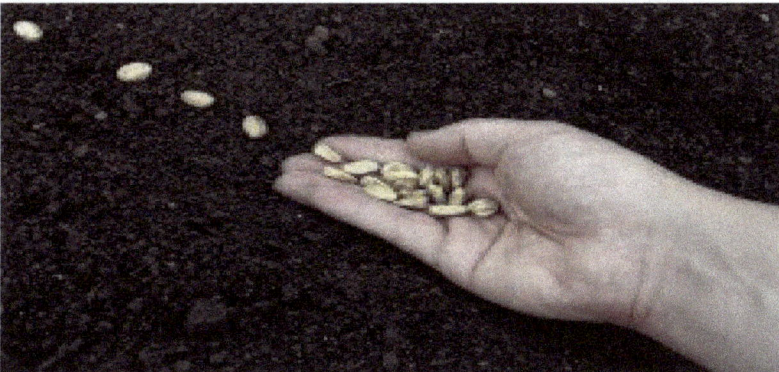

Azure/Shutterstock.com

All the building-block atoms required to build you and me are right here on Earth in the "dust" (soil), rain, air, seeds, and sunshine. The garden or field is like a shopping mall where the right numbers of the required building materials, atoms, have to be found amongst all the unneeded ones, then carried to the building site for assembly into our fruit and vegetables.

God assembles the required atoms exactly in accordance with each seed's requirements, in making our various foods.

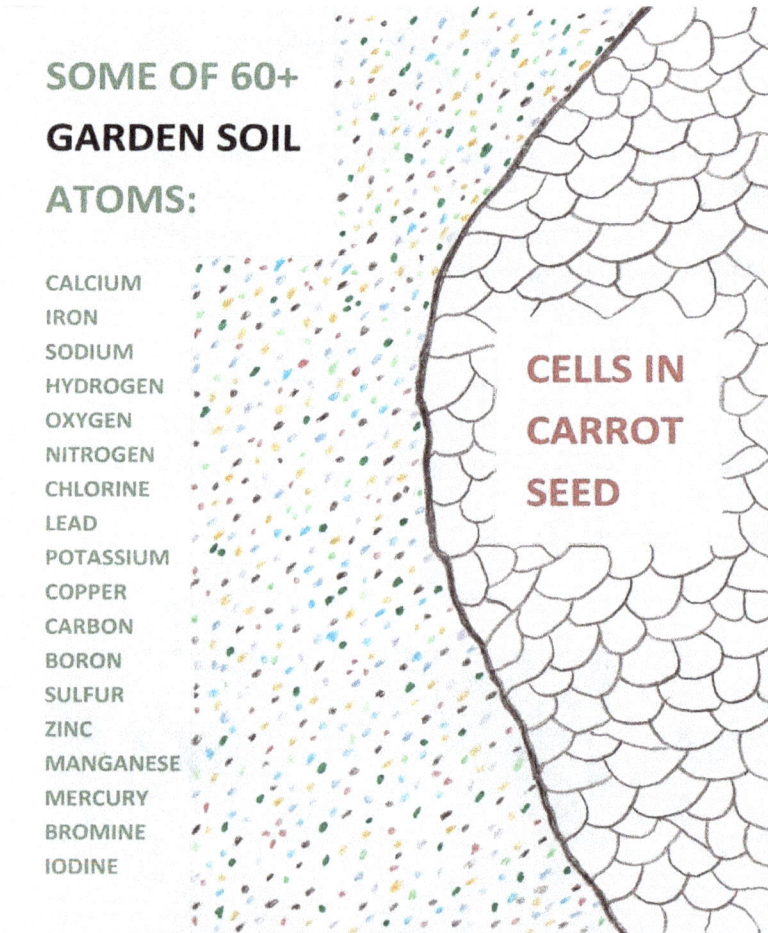

SOME OF 60+ **GARDEN SOIL** ATOMS:

CALCIUM
IRON
SODIUM
HYDROGEN
OXYGEN
NITROGEN
CHLORINE
LEAD
POTASSIUM
COPPER
CARBON
BORON
SULFUR
ZINC
MANGANESE
MERCURY
BROMINE
IODINE

CELLS IN CARROT SEED

In this simplistic diagram, the colored dots represent various elemental atoms in a typical garden's soil. They are next to a magnified image of a section of a carrot seed planted in the soil. The seed may have been dormant in a package for several years before being planted. If the gardener adds some water because he wants the carrot seed to begin "growing," these atoms must begin being moved to their proper position to build the cell's parts. The first little root hairs must be precisely built onto the seed in order to begin the carrot-building process. If you were the builder, where would you decide to begin building the root hair, and which atoms would you choose, and in what sequence?

This example gives graphic detail of the superintelligent work necessary to begin the construction of our food using some of the 60 types of atoms our body needs.

Can you imagine the sequential physical work-steps it will take to build the carrot? Only the right numbers of the right required atoms will be selected and placed to build even the first tiny root hairs. Clearly, the need for God exists to produce the design plan, and accurately assemble the correct numbers of the correct atoms for this construction project.

Our body is normally constructed of about 60 different types of elemental atoms. Besides the elements shown in the diagram, we need food containing phosphorous, magnesium, fluorine, silicon, rubidium, strontium, aluminum, cadmium, cerium, barium, tin, selenium, nickel, chromium, arsenic, cesium, molybdenum, germanium, cobalt, antimony, silver, niobium, zirconium, lanthanum, tellurium, gallium, bismuth, thallium, indium, gold, scandium, tantalum, vanadium, thorium, uranium, samarium, tungsten, beryllium, and radium.

Oxygen, carbon, hydrogen, nitrogen, calcium, phosphorous, potassium, sulfur, sodium, chlorine, and magnesium are the primary components by volume in our bodies. The rest are required in trace proportions but still important to our life and health. Determining how many atoms of each element to select and where to place them is crucial.

That process of finding and assembling the right numbers of the required atoms from our food intake has to be repeated to construct the great variety of new cells needed for our body and life.

When you understand even just a little about engineering, construction, and/or manufacturing, as well as maintenance, repair, and replacement of damaged parts, you know the importance of assembling the right materials accurately in accordance with good design plans. Precisely assembling, and fastening atoms, and precisely programming the DNA and RNA codes for the functioning of all of the highly complex cells is crucial for life in our growing foods and in us.

This two-step process of making us from "dust" is essential for our construction, sustenance, growth, maintenance, and repair. All of this amazing work cannot be performed in an unguided, random manner or left to chance. These life-giving works are performed not just for believers but also for atheists, evolutionists, and others who do not yet acknowledge this Creator who cares so much for each one of us, every second of every day.

Think of just one of our marvelously designed and built organs, like our heart, for example. If we live for 80 years, it will have to be designed, constructed, and maintained to 'beat' or 'pump' our blood about 60 times per minute x 60 minutes/hour = 3.600 times per hour x 24 hours/day = 86,400 times per day x 365 days/year = 31,536,000 times per year x 80 years = 2,522,880,000 heartbeats in our first 80 years. Quite impressive for something constructed from dust, isn't it?

How brilliantly made and carefully maintained is that piece of human machinery? We have to do our part to take care of ourselves also. God can only work with the materials we put in our mouth or breathe in.

And when we consider all our other organs that work so well for so long, we can give a little "Thank you" to God for His enormous care for us, can't we? He provides for us every day. Why would it be so reliable and constant if the motivation to provide it were not immense, loving care for us? For what other reason could it be?

Since all of this necessary work and care and much more are provided to us free of charge for our whole lifetime, it is easily understandable why we can all rightfully say, "In God We Can Trust."

No wonder many of the founders and leaders of our four nations recognized, acknowledged and consulted Him and have made Him an official part of our governance. Why is it seemingly illegal to teach our students anything about Him? This is wrong and must be changed. What we are providing here is useful science and history, not religion. **Students have the right to be taught why God is so highly recognized by their government.**

We have summarized a number of the key factors in the *"...absolute break-down of my theory* (of evolution)*",* to use Mr. Darwin's own words.

The following seven basic principles of life provide some of the reasons why a caring, all-knowing creator is required to design, construct, sustain, maintain, and repair all living entities, especially us human beings.

Seven Basic Principles of Life

Principle #1
Virtually all matter, living or not living, is constructed of atoms that do not have legs, brains, fins, or muscles to move themselves. Since atoms have no internal means to move themselves into any precise position in a cell, a capable external means is required to find, sort, select, count, grasp, and precisely place all of the right numbers of the right atoms necessary to build each cell of our food (fruit, vegetables, cereals, etc.); then, to perform a similar process selecting the right numbers of the right atoms from our digested food and placing them precisely to build each of our 40+ types of complex molecular machines for our 200+ types of cells for our body; and then to precisely position each cell type in our body, fasten it there, and hook it up properly to our blood vessels and nerve networks. Cells don't just divide. Intelligent decisions and choices have to be made constantly, e.g., where and when to change from building a bone cell to a tendon cell, then where and when to change from building tendon cells to making muscle cells, then to nerve cells, then to skin cells, and to eye cells, to ear cells, all with planned precision and in proper sequence. There are trillions of decisions, choices, selections, and assemblies to make for our life.

Every step must be performed with ultrasmart planning, care, dexterity, precision, and speed. In the English language, this phenomenally intelligent, reliable, trustworthy, and caring entity is called "God."

As evolution, by definition, has no intelligence to work with, it is now factually falsified as the true origin and cause of life and that is a very good thing for our nations. Let's get rid of this damaging deception.

Since the theory of evolution is falsified as the explanation of the origin and cause of life, it should be moved to the History Department and replaced with an accurate life science.

Principle #2

The superintelligent physical work required to build living cells, goes far beyond the parameters of possibility for the unguided processes theorized as Darwinisms.

As shown, over 4900 quadrillion correct atoms per second must be carefully selected, counted, and precisely assembled just to make replacement red blood cells for each adult person; and in the same second more than that number of atoms have to be carefully selected, counted, and precisely assembled to make the food items for each future second's new red blood cells for each person (over 10,000 quadrillion correct atoms per second).[13]

This is in addition to the phenomenal, reliable, caring physical work of constantly maintaining, repairing, and/or replacing the other approximately 80 trillion cells in each human adult body.

As evolution cannot do this enormous, intelligent work, it is falsified as the true origin and cause of life.

Principle #3

"Dead dogs don't bark," which is to say that although all the right atoms, molecules, and cells are precisely built and placed into their correct position for its eyes, ears, teeth, brain, legs, heart, lungs, paws, liver, kidneys, stomach, fir, claws, nose, and so on, **without the divine "breath of life," those atoms, molecules and cells are not going to move one millimeter.** This God-given "breath of life" is crucial to every living entity. When it is

removed, the entity's life ends. Evolution cannot provide the essential "breath of life," therefore the theory of evolution as the true origin and cause of life, is factually falsified and that is a very good thing for our nations.

Principle #4

Evolution is not a purposeful force or an intelligent agent. By definition, it has absolutely no intelligence, guidance, or plan to work with. ***However, all of these attributes plus superintelligent vision, dexterity, precision, and speed are essential to construct, grow, maintain, repair, and care for each living entity.***

As evolution is not a process with foresight capable of performing these tasks, it cannot be the cause of life, and is therefore falsified as both the origin and cause of life.

Principle #5

Mr. Darwin said his theory of evolution could "absolutely break down" if the fossil recorders did not find examples of one kind of creature gradually changing into another kind of creature (i.e. macroevolution). This would indicate that creatures do not evolve from one kind to another kind. He knew there would need to be enormous numbers of transition fossils. In his book, *On the Origin of Species,* he states, *"But just in proportion as this process of extermination has acted on an enormous scale, so must the number of intermediate varieties, which have formerly existed, be truly enormous. Why then is not every geological formation and every stratum full of such intermediate links? Geology assuredly does not reveal any such finely-graduated organic chain; and this, perhaps is the most obvious and serious objection which can be urged against my theory."* [14]

Out of the multi-millions of fossils uncovered in the earth, there should be millions of transitions, but they do not exist. For example, there are no fossils of a man with a monkey's tail. Men and monkeys still exist, yet there is not even one undisputed complete transitional ape-man creature in existence or in the fossil record.[15]

What we have found are minor changes within species such as different colors and sizes of humans, horses, cats, dogs, fish, birds, bugs, etc.

The occasional random mutations occurring between generations, that were at one time thought to be the cause of improvements in a species, actually involve a loss of DNA information. A more accurate word for these mutational changes is "devolution" or "degeneration," *never a change of one life kind to another kind; no solid evidence of macroevolution exists.*

There have been many attempts to produce images of transitions from bone fragments and there are fossils that have some characteristics similar to other kinds of creatures. However, the understanding of the enormous amount of intelligent work involved in designing and building living entities with atoms, points far more logically to a common designer and builder rather than a common ancestor.

As stated by Dr. Gary Parker, a paleontologist, biologist, and former evolutionist, *"Fossils are a great embarrassment to evolutionary theory and strong support for the concept of Creation."* [16]

The lack of transitional specimen fossils is a reassurance that evolution is factually falsified as the cause of life.

Principle #6

All living entities are built of cells containing DNA and/or RNA. DNA is like a very sophisticated, highly complex computer soft-ware program which assists in the multiple and varied functions which cells have to perform to keep a living entity alive.

Complex, intelligent, functional codes, like those in DNA, cannot be programmed without an intelligent programmer.

As evolution does not have any intelligence needed to produce complex coding, it is factually falsified as the cause of life.

Principle #7

There are many factors that must be intelligently tuned, highly regulated, and crucially consistent in order for our planet to function, and for living entities to exist. Random, uncontrolled, inconsistent conditions would quickly lead to extinction of creatures.

A few conditions under which life would not exist include:

1. If temperatures were too hot or too cold;
2. If there was insufficient water available;
3. If there was no food;
4. If there was no one to build living cells from atoms;
5. If there was no one to breathe life into these cells;
6. If there was no controlled sunlight;
7. If there was no controlled atmosphere;
8. If there was no controlled gravity;
9. If there was no controlled electricity;
10. If there was no superintelligent controller to keep all of these necessary factors (and more) in balance, life would not exist.

Fortunately for the creatures on our planet, we have a controller who reliably and consistently keeps everything necessary for food and life in balance.

As evolution, by definition, has no intelligence to fine-tune all of these essential factors, it is factually falsified as the origin and cause of life.

Essential, intelligent, physical works are required to build and maintain each living entity, however, evolution cannot perform them as, by definition, it has no intelligence to use.

1. Evolution cannot *see atoms and think of what to do with them*;
2. It cannot *find* all the necessary 'building-block' atoms;
3. It cannot *sort* the right atoms from the wrong ones for building each cell part;
4. It cannot *count* the right numbers of each type of atom for building each cell part;
5. It cannot *grasp and transport* the right atoms for building each cell part.
6. It cannot *precisely place* each atom to build each cell part;

7. It cannot *fasten* each atom in its correct place in each cell part;
8. It cannot *program* the RNA and DNA molecules as required for each cell;
9. It cannot *breathe life into* the inanimate atoms in each cell;
10. It cannot *re-sort* the atoms from our foods to build our human cells;
11. It cannot *work quickly,* or at all;
12. It cannot *build* a living entity;
13. It cannot *sustain* the life of a living entity;
14. It cannot *maintain* any entity;
15. It cannot *repair* or heal any entity;
16. It cannot *build communication systems* within living entities;
17. It cannot *fine-tune our living conditions* on our planet;
18. It cannot *build blood vessels and nerve networks* for creatures.

These are only a few of the tasks that evolution cannot perform, which are necessary for life on our planet.

Therefore, Evolution is factually falsified as the cause of life.

At the time of the founding of our nations, not all of this science was known or understood in detail by our founding fathers.

However, the need for external help with: growing crops of grains, vegetables, and fruit for food; the producing of cattle for milk and meat; fish and fowl to eat; etc., was all appreciated and understood to be intelligently, reliably, and faithfully created for the benefit of mankind.

They called this omniscient external provider, "God," just as the majority of citizens and governments in our four nations do today.

It is time to teach our students about the truth of *essential superintelligence, physical works, and awesome care* for the design, construction, sustenance, maintenance, and repair of all living entities, especially us.

What could be more obvious than the need to provide *accurate* information for our students of all ages and stages of their education?

Why should we continue to teach our future problem-solvers false information like 'Evolution' as the cause of life, then expect them to come up with the best solutions for life science problems?

If we teach them that the essentials of life just *randomly* happen and then expect them to develop the best food plans, medicines, and so on, how realistic is that on our part?

For some people, evolutionism may have seemed to be a desirable explanation as the cause for and development of living entities. However, in light of these recent discoveries in science, *essential, superintelligent, physical works with atoms* for the design, construction, maintenance, and repair of highly complex living cells and entities, i.e., "Atomic Biology," should become, by far, *the best explanation of the true cause of life.*

What we can thank evolutionists for is their thorough work in attempting to prove through all possible means that there is no need for a Creator. It seems that they have left no stone unturned in endeavoring to show another possible way that living entities could have been designed, built, sustained, maintained, and repaired without any intelligent help. *As they have performed this exhaustive search for an alternative to our Creator and have failed, it is, therefore, with ease that we can lay the 'Theory of Evolution' to rest as an unworkable philosophy for explaining the origin, cause, and complexities of Life.*

Isn't it time to return to doing science properly and follow the evidence wherever it leads? Your thoughts?

_____

_____

_____

Isn't it also time to teach truth and accuracy in science and everywhere?

_____

_____

_____

_____

_God's Style of "Evolution": – evolving a crawling worm into a
beautiful flying butterfly in a matter of days, not millions of years._

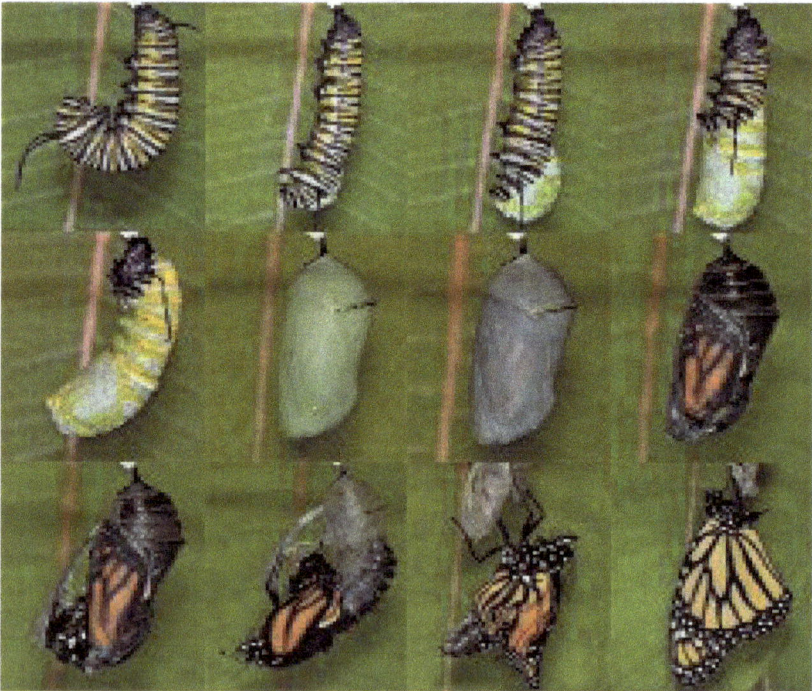

Stephen Russell Smith Photos/Shutterstock.com

Does *anyone* seriously believe that there is no intelligent work involved in this magnificent and speedy demolition and new construction work?

The Scientific Method for Verification of Factualness

"To be considered a scientific 'fact'," says Dr. Kenneth L. Currie of the Department of Geological Survey of Canada, *"a concept must pass two tests. First, it must be repeatable; that is,*

the same concatenation of circumstances always produces the same result. Second, it must be impersonal; that is, the same set of circumstances yields the same observation to different observers, or to a suitably adjusted machine." [17]

Similarly, as stated by Gary Kemper, Hallie Kemper, and Casey Luskin, *"The scientific method* (for verification of a scientific fact) *is usually described as a four-step process consisting of: 1. Observation; – 2. Hypothesis; – 3. Experiment-ation; – 4. Conclusion."* [18]

Using the Scientific Method, let's start verifying some examples of God's phenomenal work for us through this potentially new branch of God-based life science called "Atomic Biology".

VERIFICATION #1:

The superintelligent cause of life known as our Creator God, constructs our vegetables and other food plants.

Step 1. Observation

To observe the construction of plants that we can use for our own nutrition, let's choose a carrot seed, a cucumber seed, a strawberry seed, and a wheat seed and put them into an open-top glass box, like an aquarium, after we fill it three-quarters full of garden soil. Then put the seeds against the front glass about one inch from the top of the soil, so we can observe their growth. Add water and watch the superintelligent construction of the roots and foods.

The various kinds of seeds that God creates contain design plans for their unique type of living entity.

Each and every time we observe the "growth" of any entity, we are witnessing "construction" in progress. In the case of a building, all the materials plus builders' work and skills are visible. In the case of living entities for our food, the building materials are the selected atoms from the soil, water, and air. Although, they and the skills to handle them are too minute to be seen (at this time), the results of the brilliant construction work are visible.

Add a little water to the soil and watch what happens daily over the next few weeks. A good magnifying glass will make it more interesting.

Better yet, we could use a magnifying video camera that takes a picture about every fifteen minutes to record the construction of each type of food plant.

Observe the gradual assembly of atoms into tiny root hairs being built onto each seed using atoms from the soil, water, air, and some from the seed. Although we are not able to actually see the individual atoms being sorted, selected, grasped, counted, and precisely placed in each cell, we know this has to be happening by seeing the *results* of this intelligent physical work, the construction progress, and the finished products, complete with the vitamins, minerals and other nutrients built in for us.

The majority of the atoms in our plants include carbon, hydrogen, nitrogen, oxygen, sodium, calcium, iron, potassium, phosphorus, and smaller quantities of a large variety of other elemental atoms shown on pages 92-93.

In a few days, we observe the beginning of the construction of the roots and bodies or stems of each plant. The right numbers of the right building-block atoms are being found at the right time in the soil and water, then sorted, selected, grasped, counted, conducted in through the roots, and precisely assembled into the right type of cells needed for the next steps in the plant's progressive, critical-path construction. Various colors are added to the parts of the plants as the builder desires, always including some green for the chlorophyll that helps to gather energy and other aid from the sunlight, or an alternate light.

We can observe each food plant being reliably built according to its seed type and design, all the way up to maturity, complete with more seeds. Carrots are usually harvested before their seeds are constructed, but some are allowed to go on to the seed construction stage.

A single wheat stock can be built with 20, 40, or more seeds that are normally made into cereal or flour for our bread or other baked goods.

We can repeat endlessly the planting of seeds and observing the building of food plants, as others have for millennia, with the same life-sustaining nutrients built in by the Builder.

Step 2. Hypothesis

We know that *atoms have <u>no internal means</u> or intelligence to move themselves precisely* into their correct place in each cell. Therefore, <u>*they require an intelligent external means*</u> to grasp the correct atoms, select, count, and assemble them quickly, and fasten them precisely and reliably according to an extremely complex and sophisticated plan.

Remembering that evolution has no intelligence, and that our best human intelligence using sophisticated equipment is not sufficient to come anywhere close to constructing even one small, living, functional molecular machine for a cell, we have thus shown that a *greater intelligence than we have is essential to design and build living entities.*

Because superintelligence is required by this external agent, the best explanation for the cause of life is to credit our Creator, the God of our nations, for this phenomenal, life-giving, physical work with atoms. This is part of what makes Him, "God."

Step 3. Experimentation

We can experiment repeatedly by planting more seeds, from tiny mustard seeds to larger watermelon seeds, to grow foods.

The planting and growing of seeds can be repeated endlessly as has been performed for millennia with the same reliable, life-sustaining nourishment installed by the Builder.

One advantage of planting seeds in a glass case is that we can observe at least part of the construction of each type of plant, starting with its first tiny roots.

Imagine the enormous amount of other work needed to build enough food for all the eight billion people on Earth every day. God does build enough for everyone, but we don't share it with others as well as we could and should.

In the early 1990's, when government debts were soaring, I was working on a project to find ways of increasing government efficiency. One of my relatives in South Africa sent me some information that they gave to their poor and needy people instead of money. It was one double-sided page of instructions on how to grow enough food for one person, on a piece of ground the size of a door (3 feet by 7 feet)! Diagrams showed how to plant various seeds, harvest the vegetables and fruit when ready, return leaves and peelings to the ground along with more seeds, and keep rotating the process. This works best in climates with year-round growing seasons, but with suitable green boxes, growing time can be extended anywhere.

Experiments that involve planting various kinds of seeds and observing them being built precisely and carefully using the right atoms from the soil, air, and water, into each respective kind of plants, are repeatable and impersonal – the two requirements for verifying factualness.

Step 4. Conclusion

The best explanation for the origin and development of living cells and entities is that superintelligent physical work with atoms is essential to design, construct, sustain, and maintain each one.

VERIFICATION #2:

No construction of food plants is possible without the supreme-minded cause known as our Creator God and the seeds He has designed and built.

Step 1. Observation

If we want to observe the construction of some food plants *without God's help*, we cannot use seeds.

Use the same glass container and soil from Verification #1 and add water.

No food plant will grow.

There are millions of microbes (microscopic living entities) in every cubic foot of garden soil. There may be some seeds for some kinds of plant life in the soil that will grow, but where there were no food seeds planted, no food plants grow.

Step 2. Hypothesis

Regardless of how many times this experiment is repeated and by whom, no food plants will ever grow unless food seeds are planted, formally or informally.

Seeds may be *altered* through tampering by scientists, but not *created* by them.

Step 3. Experimentation

Even using the best, clean garden soil, the best fertilizers, and the best water and air available, no matter how carefully the fertilizing and watering is done, no food plants are built without the planting of God-built seeds.

Step 4. Conclusion

Regardless of how many times this experiment is repeated and by whomsoever, no food plants will ever 'grow' unless seeds are planted. This satisfies the tests of repeatability and impersonal results, i.e., the same result over and over for any observer. It also passes the test of reason.

Our accumulated research regarding the phenomenal amount of superintelligent physical work with atoms that must be performed to build, sustain, and maintain any food plant, and any one of us humans, is one of the most compelling rationales that eliminates the possibility of an unguided or unintelligent process as the designer, builder, and maintainer of living entities.

Until proven otherwise, the best explanation for the origin and cause of life in all living entities is the enormous amount of superintelligent, physical work with atoms required for the design, construction, and ongoing sustenance and maintenance of each cell in each living entity, (i.e. "Atomic Biology").

Quotable Quotes from Significant Scientists:

1. "Is it really credible that random processes could have constructed a reality, the smallest element of which – a functional protein

or gene – is complex beyond...anything produced by the intelligence of man?" [19]

> Michael Denton, biological research scientist and M.D.

2. *"At that moment, when the RNA/DNA system became understood, the debate between Evolutionists and Creationists should have come to a screeching halt."* [20]

> I. L. Cohen, archaeologist and mathematician

3. *"The likelihood of the formation of life from inanimate matter* [without intelligent help] *is one in a number with 40,000 noughts (zeroes) after it...It is big enough to bury Darwin and the whole theory of evolution."* [21]

> Sir Fred Hoyle and Chandra Wickramaisinghe,
> astronomers, physicists, and mathematicians.

4. *"An intelligible communication via radio signal from some distant galaxy would be widely hailed as evidence of an intelligent source. Why then doesn't the message sequence on the DNA molecule also constitute prima facie evidence for an intelligent source?"* [22]

Charles B. Thaxton, Walter L. Bradley, Roger L Olsen, chemists

5. *"That organic evolution could account for the complex forms of life in the past and the present has long since been abandoned by men who grasp the importance of the DNA genetic code."* [23] John Grebe, chemist

6. *"From the claims made for Neo-Darwinism one could easily get the impression that it has made great progress towards explaining Evolution... In fact, quite the reverse is true."* [24]

Peter T. Saunders, mathematician, and Mae-Wan Ho, geneticist

7. *"We have to admit that there is nothing in the geological records that runs contrary to the view of the conservative creationists, that God created each species."* [25]

Edmund Ambrose, evolutionist, cell biologist

8. *"There is no recorded experiment in the history of science that contradicts the second law (of thermodynamics) or its corollaries...".*[26]

G. Hatsopoulous and E. Gyftopoulos, physicists

(The second law of thermodynamics shows that everything left unmaintained by an external intelligence, tends to deteriorate).

9 *"Of all the statements that have been made with respect to theories on the origin of life, the statement that the Second Law of Thermodynamics poses no problem for an evolutionary origin of life is the most absurd...."* [27] Duane Gish, biochemist.

10. *"The Evolutionist thesis has become more stringently unthinkable than ever before..."* [28]

Wolfgang Smith, physicist and mathematician

11. *"As is now well known, most fossil species appear instantaneously in the fossil record."* [29]

Tom Kemp, curator of Zoological Collections at Oxford U.

12. *"Evolution requires intermediate forms between species and paleontology does not provide them."* [30]

David Kitts, paleontologist and evolutionist

13. *"The preservation of numerous soft-bodied Cambrian animals as well as Precambrian embryos and micro-organisms undermines the idea of an extensive period of undetected soft-bodied evolution. In addition, the claim that exclusively soft-bodied ancestors preceded the hard-bodied Cambrian forms remains anatomically implausible."* [31]

Stephen C. Meyer, science philosopher

14. *"A growing number of respectable scientists are defecting from the evolutionist camp, moreover, for the most part these "experts" have abandoned Darwinism, not on the basis of religious faith or biblical persuasions, but on strictly scientific grounds."* [32]   -- Wolfgang Smith, physicist.

15. *"It is the sheer universality of perfection, the fact that every-where we look, to whatever depth we look, we find an elegance and ingenuity of an absolute transcending quality which so mitigates against the idea of chance."* [33]
Michael Denton, biological research scientist and medical doctor.

16. *"The theory of evolution...will be one of the great jokes in the history books of the future. Posterity will marvel that so flimsy and dubious an hypothesis could be accepted with the incredible credulity that it has."* [34]
Malcolm Muggeridge, philosopher

17. *"Human DNA is like a computer program but far, far more advanced than any software we've ever created."* [35]
Bill Gates, founder of Microsoft

18. *"...the amount of information that could be stored in a pinhead's volume of DNA is staggering. ... a pinhead of DNA would have the equivalent information of a pile of CD's 1,000 miles high, or 40 million times as much as a 100-gigabyte hard drive."* [36]
Jonathan Sarfati, physical chemist

19. *"No undirected physical or chemical process has ever demonstrated the capacity to produce specified information starting from purely physical or chemical precursors. For this reason, chemical evolutionary theories have failed to solve the mystery of the origin of first life—a claim that few mainstream evolutionary theorists now dispute."* [37]
Stephen C. Meyer, science philosopher

20. *"It is certainly true that a machine carefully made by a craftsman reflects the existence of its creator. It would be foolish to suggest that time and chance could make a computer or a microwave oven, or that the individual parts could form themselves into these complex mechanisms.... Yet life is far, far more complex than any man-made machine."* [38]

   Paul S. Taylor, science author and motion picture producer

21. *"Any suppression which undermines and destroys that very foundation on which scientific methodology and research was erected, evolutionist or otherwise, cannot and must not be allowed to flourish. ...It is a confrontation between scientific objectivity and ingrained prejudice. ...In the final analysis, objective scientific analysis has to prevail – no matter what the final result is – no matter how many time-honored idols have to be discarded in the process....*

   It is not the duty of science to defend the theory of evolution, and stick by it to the bitter end – no matter what illogical and unsupported conclusions it offers... If in the process of impartial scientific logic, they find that creation by outside superintelligence is the solution to our quandary, then let's cut the umbilical cord that tied us down to Darwin for such a long time. It is choking us and holding us back.

   *...Every single concept advanced by the theory of evolution (and amended thereafter) is imaginary as it is not supported by the scientifically established facts of microbiology, fossils, and mathematical probability concepts. Darwin was wrong. ... **The theory of evolution may be the worst mistake made in science.**"* [39] (emphasis added)

   I. L. Cohen, archaeologist and mathematician

If the theory of evolution cannot provide an explanation of how it performs the essential superintelligent work of finding the right atoms in the soil, air, and water to construct all the cell parts required to build any vegetable or fruit; how it intelligently selects the right atoms from the wrong ones; how it counts the right numbers of each correct type of atoms for each cell part; how it *grasps these right numbers of right atoms and places them precisely and fastens them securely and properly to build each cell part; how it makes and properly sequences the billions of bases for the DNA and RNA in foods and creatures, how it constructs the molecular machines and other crucial complex parts in each cell; how it adds the essential "breath of life" to make each cell live and function; and how it can precisely handle over 4900 quadrillion right atoms per second in each adult, just to build his or her replacement red blood cells as just one part of our life support; and how this can all be done with no intelligence or guidance, **then the theory of evolution should be fully classified as falsified.***

If Darwinism/Neo-Darwinism/macroevolution do not work, are incorrect, falsified, and misleading, by what justification should they continue to be taught?   This is a serious question for our scientists, our educators, our leaders, parents, students, and the Supreme Court of the USA.

We all receive an immense amount of God's physical work and care every second of every day.   It is time to make the change and bring understanding and appreciation of our Creator, the God of our governments, back to our classrooms.

Does He have the right to be upset with people that disrespect Him and show no gratitude for His enormous works for them every second of every day?

Perhaps He will be more upset with those educators who purposefully withhold the Truth about His immense works for everyone.

What do you think? _____

_____

_____

Applications for Life.

1. How much intelligence does 'evolution' have, and how do we know this? _____

_____

2. Do humans have enough intelligence to build the molecular machines for cells, and how do we know this? _____

_____

_____

3. What are the names of four of the scientists who have shown that mankind cannot build the molecular machines for a living cell?_____

_____

4. Do you think it is important to know the correct cause of life, and why? _____

_____

5. Do you think it is proper that teachers and professors in secular schools and colleges are forced to teach that only 'evolution' is the cause of life, and why? _____

_____

6. Who said, "The theory of evolution may be the worst mistake made in science." _____

7. How many "Basic Principles For Life" does this chapter show?

_____

8. What "Essential, intelligent, physical works" for building and maintaining each living entity are shown in this chapter and why can 'evolution' not perform them? _____

_____

_____

9. In the list of "Quotable Quotes from Significant Scientists," which three quotes do you like the most (by number) and why?

_____

_____

_____

_____

_____

_____

References and Notes:

[1] Hoyle, Sir Fred and Chandra Wickramasinghe, *Evolution from Space,* J. M. Dent & Sons, London, England, 1981, p. 148.

[2] Meyer, Stephen C., *Signature in the Cell,* Harper Collins, New York, NY, 2009, p. 201.

[3] Darwin, Charles, *On the Origin of Species by Means of Natural Selection,* 1st edition, John Murray, London, England, 1859, p.189, available online from Darwin-online.org.uk.

[4] Ibid., p. 186.

[5] Ibid., p. 189.

[6] Darwin, Charles, in a letter to Asa Gray (April 3, 1860), as

cited in Norman MacBeth's *Darwin Retried: An Appeal To Reason*, Gambit Publications Ltd., Boston, MA, 1971, p. 101.

[7] *A Scientific Dissent from Darwinism,*
www.dissentfromdarwin.com; accessed May 20, 2014.

[8] Ruloff, W., J. Sullivan, Logan Craft (Producers), &
N. Frankowski, (Director), *Expelled: No Intelligence Allowed,*
DVD, Premise Media Corporation & Rampant Films, 2008.

[9] Luskin, C., "Bullies-r-us: how 'freethought oasis' threatened 'disruption' and pressured a college into cancelling intelligent design course," 10 December, 2013, *Evolution News and Views,* www.evolutionnews.org/2013/12/freethought-oasisbullies079991.html; accessed May 20, 2014.

[10] Bergman, J., *Slaughter of the Dissidents: The Shocking Truth About Killing the Careers of Darwin Doubters*; Leafcutter Press, Southworth, WA, 2012; *Silencing the Darwin Skeptics,* Leafcutter Press, Southworth, WA, 2016; and *Censoring the Darwin Skeptics, How Belief in Evolution is Enforced by Eliminating Dissidents*, Leafcutter Press, Southworth, WA,'18

[11] Lewontin, R., *Billions and Billions of Demons*, The New York Review of Books, New York, NY, 9 January, 1997.

[12] Rogers, T., (Producer), and Woodyard, J. (Music Director), *"Goodbye, Evolution,"* CD, Creation Studios, Canada, 2009.

[13] Pallister, C. J., *Haematology: Biomedical Science Explained,* Butterworth-Heinemann, Burlington, MA, 1999. He states that an average 70 kg adult male produces *(or has produced for him)* about 2,300,000 red blood cells every second.

Tortora, G. J., *Principles of Anatomy and Physiology,* John Wiley & Sons, New York, NY, 2008. He states that there are approximately 280,000,000 molecules of hemoglobin per red blood cell.

Perutz, Max, *Science Is Not a Quiet Life: Unraveling the*

Atomic Mechanism of Hemoglobin, World Scientific, Hackensack, NJ, 1997. He states that each hemoglobin molecule contains approximately 10,000 atoms.

If you do the math, you will find that the number of atoms required to be sorted from our eaten food, then selected, counted, grasped, and assembled into new red blood cells and delivered into our bloodstream is approximately 2,300,000 x 280,000,000 x 10,000 = 6,440,000,000,000,000,000 (6,440 quadrillion) atoms every second of every day.

That approximate number is required for each average body every second of every day just for replacement red blood cells (based on a 70 kilo [154 lb.] male as average). We have conservatively used the figure of "over 4,900 quadrillion atoms per second" to include each of virtually all adults in the world. Rogers, Thomas, Jerry Bergman, Graham McLennan, (this book).

[14] Darwin, Charles, *On the Origin of Species by Means of Natural Selection,* 1st edition, John Murray, London, England, 1859, p. 280; available online from Darwin-online.org.uk.

[15] Bergman, Jerry, Peter Line, and Jeffrey Tomkins, *Apes as Ancestors: Examining the Claims About Human Evolution,* Bartlett Publishing, Tulsa, OK., 2020.

[16] Parker, Gary, in Paul S. Taylor's *Origins Answer Book,* 4th Edition, Eden Productions, Mesa, Arizona, 1993, p. 103.

[17] Currie, Kenneth L., "Uniformity, Uniformitarianism, and the Foundations of Science" in Paul A. Zimmerman's *Rock Strata and the Bible Record,* Concordia Publishing House, St. Louis, MO, 1970, p. 40.

[18] Kemper, Gary, Hallie Kemper, and Casey Luskin, *Discovering Intelligent Design: A Journey Into The Scientific Evidence,* Discovery Institute Press, Seattle, WA, 2013, p.221.

[19] Denton, Michael, *Evolution: A Theory in Crisis,* Burnett Books, London, England, 1985, p. 342.

[20] Cohen, I.L., *Darwin Was Wrong—A Study In Probabilities,* New Research Publications, New York, NY, 1984, p. 5.

[21] Hoyle, Sir Fred, and Chandra Wickramasinghe, *Evolution From Space*, Aldine House, London, England, 1981, p. 149.

[22] Thaxton, Charles B., Walter L. Bradley, and Roger L. Olsen, *The Mystery Of Life's Origin: Reassessing Current Theories,* Philosophical Library, New York, NY, 1984, pp. 211-212.

[23] Grebe, John J., *"DNA Complexity Points to Divine Design,"* Science & Scripture, vol. 3, no. 3, p. 20, Creation Science Research Center, San Diego, CA, 1973.

[24] Saunders, Peter and Mae-Wan Ho, *"Is Neo-Darwinism Falsifiable? And Does It Matter?"* Nature and System, vol. 4, no. 4, December 1982, Tucson, AZ, p. 191.

[25] Ambrose, Edmund J., *The Nature and Origin of the Biological World,* John Wiley & Sons, New York, NY, 1982, p.164

[26] Hatsopoulous, G. N. and E.P. Gyftopoulos, *Deductive Quantum Thermodynamics,* Mono Book Corporation, Baltimore, MA, 1970, p. 78.

[27] Gish, Duane, *"A Consistent Christian Scientific View of the Origin of Life,"* Creation Research Society Quarterly, vol. 15, no. 4, March 1979, pp.186, 199.

[28] Smith, Wolfgang, *Teilhardism and the New Religion: A Thorough Analysis of the Teachings of Pierre Teilhard de Chardin*, Tan Books and Publishers, Rockford, IL, 1988, p. 8.

[29] Kemp, Tom, "A Fresh Look at the Fossil Record," *New Scientist,* vol. 108, no. 1485, December 1985, p. 66.

30 Kitts, David B., "Paleontology and Evolutionary Theory," *Evolution,* vol. 28, September 1974, p. 467.

31 Meyer, Stephen C., *Darwin's Doubt: The Explosive Origin Of Animal Life,* Harper-Collins Publishers, New York, NY, 2013, p. 105.

32 Smith, J. Wolfgang, 1988, *Teilhardism and the New Religion: A Thorough Analysis of the Teachings of Pierre Teilhard de Chardin,* Tan Books and Publishers, Rockford, IL., p. 248.

33 Denton, Michael, *Evolution: A Theory In Crisis,* Adler & Adler Publishers, Bethesda, MD, 1986, p. 342.

34 Muggeridge, Malcolm, *Pascal Lectures,* University of Waterloo, Waterloo, ON, Canada, 1978.

35 Gates, Bill, Nathan Myhrvold, and Peter Rinearson, *The Road Ahead: Completely Revised and Up-To-Date,* Penguin Books, New York, NY, 1996, p. 228.

36 Sarfati, Jonathan, *Refuting Evolution,* Fourth Edition, Creation Ministries International, Eight Mile Plains, QLD, Australia, 2008, p. 121.

37 Meyer, Stephen C., *Darwin's Doubt: The Explosive Origin Of Animal Life,* Harper-Collins Publishers, New York, NY, 2013, p. iv.

38 Taylor, Paul S., *The Illustrated Origins Answer Book,* Fourth Edition, Eden Productions, Mesa, AZ, 1993, pp. 25–26.

39 Cohen, I.L., *Darwin Was Wrong—A Study in Probabilities,* New Research Publications, Greendale, NY, 1984, pp. 209-210.

Part II:

Bringing the God of Our Nation Back to Our Students as the True Creator, Provider, and Maintainer of Their Life, 24/7.

Chapter 8

Some Persons Dislike Their Concept of God

Even Richard Dawkins, who has often spoken for the atheists of the world, has recently admitted that the loss of the influence of Christianity would be bad for society.[1] **He also now refers to himself as a "cultural Christian."** [2]

When you read the first few quotes at the beginning of Chapter 1, you may be surprised to learn that Darwin was probably a believer in our Creator at the time he wrote his *Origins* book. His wife, Emma Darwin, who edited *Origins,* certainly was.

However, Darwin's work was used as a destructive influence against God, and nothing good ever came from that scenario.

Darwin's theory has been used in an effort to totally remove our Creator, the God of our nation, from public education. This ploy has been widely used in the last few decades, to the detriment, not only to our students, but also to our governments and society in general.

The resulting moral decline and increase in anxiety, depression, and hopelessness, have led to increasing illegal drug use with all of its degenerative effects including overdose deaths, suicides, crime to obtain addiction supplies, irresponsibility, higher costs to taxpayers for policing, emergency services, medical costs, and family heartaches.

Darwin's theory of evolution has been modified over the years, mainly by atheists who saw this as an opportunity to produce a 'theory' of a totally ungodly cause of life, namely "evolution."

To the unbeliever, the written word of the God of our nations, the Holy Bible, might seem like foolishness. There are aspects of this position that might seem reasonable if you consider the following examples:

1. We cannot see God in person (except for the 33 years when Jesus was on Earth).

2. His voice is not often audible to humans. Relatively few people have heard God's voice. However, there have been many credible reports of people hearing audible words from God at significant times, such as His audible warning at times of imminent danger.

3. Some find miracles, including those arranged by God, hard to accept.

4. It can seem foolish to believe in something by "faith" (although belief in evolution requires far more faith than belief in our Creator).

Since belief in evolution as the origin and cause of life, knowing how intelligently designed and complex life is, requires immense faith, this makes evolution as much of a religion as any other belief requiring faith.

Many people dislike their idea of God for various other reasons:

5. They may have been offended or hurt by someone claiming to be a Godly person or someone attending a church. Most of us have heard stories about adults abusing children in some church-related setting. This is a truly disgusting action of tempted pretenders.

In His Bible, God says that it would be better for a person to have a millstone placed around his neck and be flung into the sea, than to harm one of His little ones. He says that He judges offenders after the end of their life on Earth and sometimes before.

We have to understand that going to a church does not make anyone a Godly person any more than standing in a garage makes them a car.

Don't blame God or Jesus for what people do wrong, even if they are pretending to be Christians. True Christians try to do what they believe Jesus would do in various circumstances. But we are never perfect.

6. Some people do not like their concept of God because He seems like an intruder who watches every move they make, including, perhaps, some moves they may not want watched.

7.   They know some churchgoers who are imperfect (which includes all of us); some do bad things like anybody else, or worse, and don't stop (they are pretenders, not true Christians who "walk the walk").

8.   Some people have not found reasons to believe in God yet.

An important objective of this book is to show the reader just how much our Creator, God, cares for each one of us and how hard He works providing for our lives every second of every day.

If you ever feel you are at "rock bottom," remember: "Jesus is the 'Rock' at the bottom" and He can help you up.

Here are a few thoughts that might be helpful for those who have trouble believing there exists a Creator God who cares for us immensely, and who proves this by His enormous works in providing life, food, and beautiful things for us to enjoy.

Regarding Point 1 above, it is true that we cannot see God. However, many things that exist cannot be seen. Here are a few examples:
i.   We cannot see the wind, yet it is easy to experience its effects on trees, flowers, clouds, and us;
ii.   We cannot see gravity, but we know it is there because if we drop something denser than a helium balloon, it falls downward;
iii.   We cannot see the individual atoms and molecules we are built with but we know scientifically they are there;
iv.   We cannot see warmth from the Sun but we can certainly feel it on a summer day;
v.   We cannot see love but we instinctively feel it emotionally when it is close to us.

Regarding Point 2, it is true that relatively few people have heard God's voice, however, there have been many reports of hearing audible words from God at significant times such as His audible warning at times of imminent danger while driving, boating, and so on.

Far more significant are the large numbers of people who experience answers to their prayers to God. No doubt, the inteligent people that pray privately and publicly, would not do so if they believed it was not a useful and effective exercise.

In my studies about God and His Word, I have learned and experienced that there are four separate types of answers to prayers. All these types begin with 'D':

i. First is the *Direct* answer, which comes while you are praying, or very shortly thereafter. For example, I have several times prayed to God for His help in finding small items when I have become frustrated in searching for them, and before I have finished praying the requests, I was given the exact locations.

ii. Second is the *Delayed* answer which comes after days, weeks, months, or even years of starting the prayer request. This type of answer often comes for those who have been praying for a spouse, the blessing of a baby child, for a special job, etc. For example, I prayed to God for several years for a career in His service, and finally it came. It is working on this project of developing and implementing this God-based life science of Atomic Biology.

iii. Third is the *Different* answer whereby you pray for something in particular but receive something else. Some young people might pray for a close relationship with a particular person, and that does not occur; instead, another individual, often one more compatible, does become their special boyfriend or girlfriend.

iv. Fourth is the *Denied* answer which often happens because God knows what is best for us. He can deny the item we prayed for but will often send something better for us.

In general, those who believe in God will probably say that they receive messages and advice from Him most often while reading or hearing His Word as written in the Bible.

Regarding Point 3, God's "miracles" are well documented in many modern books, as well as in the Bible. Most people who have received them, probably give God the credit. I remember one of the first "miracle healings" that I played a small part in as a fairly new believer at age 55: Katherine, a young mother of three young children, had a very painful shoulder and could not move her right hand and arm away from her side without severe pain. Her brother came to me and three others and asked if we would pray to God to heal her shoulder. After all, Katherine had to be able to handle her three children. So we each laid one of our hands on her back or shoulders and prayed for her healing for about two minutes. Then the other four people just left. So, as a new believer, I asked, "Did that help any, Kathy?" Well, she lifted her arm right up straight over her head without any pain at all! "Praise the Lord!" I said. This was exciting for me as I had not seen up close and personal – an instant healing like this before.

Regarding Point 4, although believing in something by faith might not seem very scientific, I have found that people generally have reasons for doing what they do and believing what they believe. Part of the objective of this book is to provide solid reasons to believe and have faith in our Creator God – scientific evidence here and now which can solidify our faith.

I agree with the message in the title of a 2004 book by Norman Geisler and Frank Turek, *I Don't Have Enough FAITH to Be an ATHEIST.* Knowing how highly complex, precisely built, reliably provided, and finely tuned virtually all necessities for Life are, including our grown foods, believing they could just happen with no intelligent input takes incredible faith.

Regarding Point 5, we have to remember that God is <u>not</u> the church and people are not God. We all have an enemy within us who will tempt us to do bad or even evil deeds. This is Satan of whom you have probably heard but might not understand. Satan is bright, evil, powerful, persuasive, and in competition with God for our attention. He is far smarter and stronger than we are on our own. He is very subtle and can make things that are bad for us, look good and attractive for a little while. For example, to many he will say things like, "Try a little of this crystal meth…you will feel fantastic!" And shortly after, many become trapped in one of the ugliest addictions known. And, of course, the use of fentanyl can be absolutely deadly.

In Greater Vancouver (British Columbia, Canada) alone, we now lose an average of six people per day to drug overdoses in addition to all the expensive emergency rescues.

Satan tries to lure each one of us into one of his traps. He delights in picking on people in churches to win them to his flock and make the Christian Church, which is often considered a house of God, to look bad or even disgusting.

We have to remember that we cannot blame God, or His Son Jesus, for what people do wrong.

Regarding Point 6, God will not normally prevent anyone from doing anything, and He does not report to anyone (although it seems some mothers get information on what their kids are doing wrong without seeing it!). But because He has so much work to do within each of us, including sustaining us, maintaining us, repairing, and replacing our worn-out cells with the new ones He has built for us, including brain cells, He just has to be there. He might warn us not to do something through our conscience, but He gives us the freedom to choose what we do.

Regarding Point 7, it is true that some churchgoers choose to do evil, however, it is not God's will or teaching that directs their choices.

Remember, we should not judge God or Jesus by what people do. He works phenomenally hard to provide and care for our Life, along with wonderful things for us to enjoy, including beautiful birds, flowers, fish, animals, good friends, and pets. God tries to teach us how to have a joyful life, avoid wrong choices, and to help others.

Regarding Point 8, it is true that some people do not believe in the existence of God, and others do not want to believe in His existence. After reading this book, they will have several good scientific reasons to understand and appreciate His existence, especially with this knowledge regarding the caring work that He performs reliably for each one of us every second of every day.

Does God *deserve* our appreciation for all His work for us? What do you think? _____

But Where Do Most Of Our Troubles Come From?
Exposing Subtle Satan's Powerful Ploy:

It is almost past time to sit up and take serious notice of Satan as Public Enemy #1.

One of his big and obvious goals is to destroy the belief of all believers in our Creator, and he is getting very good at this.

His favorite dark deed is to separate people, including students, from their belief and gratitude for their Creator's care.

An open and honest evolutionary biologist at Harvard, Professor Richard Lewontin, shed some revealing light onto the enforced exclusive teaching of "evolution" as both the origin and only cause of life, stating, *"We take the side of* (evolutionary) *science in spite of the patent absurdity of some of its constructs, in spite of its failure to fulfill many of its extravagant promises of health and life, in spite of the tolerance of the scientific community for unsubstantiated just-so stories, because we have a prior commitment, a commitment to materialism. It is not that the methods and institutions of science somehow compel us to accept a material explanation of the phenomenal world, but, on the contrary, that we are forced by our a priori adherence to material causes to create an apparatus of investigation and a set of concepts that produce material explanations, no matter how counter-intuitive, no matter how mystifying to the uninitiated. Moreover, that materialism is absolute, for we cannot allow a Divine Foot in the door."* [2] (Emphasis added).

What major problems does this statement reveal? First, what is being called the "science" of evolution is obviously anti-science as it disallows scientific explanations for Life to be taught.

For the good of our ongoing Society, we have to bring Truth for Life Education and God's advice to the forefront and make them available to our students.

The current accumulated effect is that for so many in our society, their moral compass is gone, their gratitude for God's foods and their Life, is virtually non-existent, and confusion over their personal identity is depressing many. They have not been given knowledge of the enormous work and care that their Creator provides for them, nor the wisdom for joyful living that He offers through His beneficial Word, the Bible.

He can help us resist the harmful temptations that Satan wants to use to trap us into addictions and many other troubles.

Applications for Life

1. What is your opinion about God? _____

_____

_____

2. Have you ever thought about how your food is made reliably from the dust of gardens, fields, and orchards?

_____

_____

3. If you are not familiar with the wise advice available in the Bible, would you read a few Proverbs?

_____

4. When you are tempted to do something that can have harmful consequences for you, can you remember to ask God, your Creator and provider, to help you resist?

_____

References and Notes

[1]https://www.breitbart.com/national-security/2016/01/12/professional-atheist-dawkins-says-christianity-bulwark-against-something-worse/

[2] Hobson, T., *Is Richard Dawkins A Christian?* spectator.co.uk, April 2, 2024.

[3] Lewontin, R., *Billions and Billions of Demons*, The New York Review of Books, New York, NY, 9 January, 1997.

Chapter 9

A Fresh Introduction to the Scientific God of Our Nations

Evidence is growing that most sciences are, at the core, studies of the works of our Creator.

Since the majority of the adult citizens in the four nations we are discussing already believe in God, only more details are needed for them. But to help those who have little knowledge of their Creator, we provide basic information regarding the enormous amount of work and care He performs for each one of us every second of every day.

A little boy, who was probably speaking for many of us, once said, "I want to see God with skin on!" And another story representing the mindset of many, said, "I'm from Missouri ... SHOW ME !"

For the latter, we are endeavoring to show ways to verify God's presence by showing visible signs of His works and care for each of us every second of every day.

Let us eliminate what we are not talking about, i.e. the mythical Greek, Roman, Egyptian, or other mythological gods.

We are referring to the Triune Creator God of the Holy Bible who is highly recognized and acknowledged by the governments of the United States, the United Kingdom, Australia, and Canada, as well as other national, state, provincial, county, and municipal governments. (See Chapters 10, 11, 12, and 13).

This Bible is the 'Manufacturer's Manual for Operators (us)'. As with other operator's manuals, its purpose is to supply advice for the user's maximum benefit.

God's guidance has always been available for the governments of these nations, and for the citizens who desire His counsel. Details that, in the past, have not been clarified, are those showing the enormous amount of *careful physical work* He performs for everybody, including atheists and evolutionists, every second of every day.

How do we know it is our Creator God who is doing all of this phenomenal work?

First, we analyzed the physical work *required* to build every morsel of our food, i.e., each vegetable, fruit, kernel of grain, etc. from the dirt.

Then we analyzed the even more brilliant essential work required to assemble our cells using the atoms from our food to build living cell parts, construct, fasten, and hook up each one of our cells to create, sustain, and maintain *us*.

Each part of these 200+ various cells is made of the required numbers of the correct atoms, and we know that atoms lack an *internal* means to move themselves into precise positions in each cell. Therefore, a superintelligent, dexterous, precise, *external* agent is required to do this work. Millions of decisions, choices, and brilliant assembly configurations with atoms must be performed at each cell construction site.

We have investigated a portion of the work that we know requires *unique vision* to find in the soil, air, and water the right numbers of the required atom types necessary for the building blocks of every fruit and vegetable, every cell for the roots, leaves, skin, etc. Then we know that superintelligent *dexterity* is required to place each atom carefully into each cell part the Builder is creating for our food. Then, after we have consumed the food He constructed for us, more *superintelligent work* must be performed to fasten each correct atom for each molecule for each different part of each complex cell part required for the construction, sustenance, growth, maintenance, and repair of our bodies, every second of every day.

Humans, with all our accumulated scientific knowledge and sophisticated equipment, have verified over the last seventy years, that we cannot make even one significant part of a living cell, using atoms and given any length of time.

We know, therefore, that to accomplish the enormous amount of brilliant works essential to build entire food cells and human cells, an all-wise source is required. Building each cell part using inanimate atoms is ultrasmart enough; however, without adding *the energizing "breath of life,"* no cell or entity can live or function. When this is removed, the cell or entity dies.

The production of our food, as one example, has been acknowledged for centuries as seemingly miraculous, and long before these details were understood, God was acknowledged as the brilliant, omniscient Producer.

Governments have provided a special day of appreciation for the enormous work that God does for us all, and that is, of course, Thanksgiving Day, or simply Thanksgiving.

To understand even a very small portion of the amazing creative *work* that has to be performed for us by our Creator, let's look at the following example.

If we desire to build a new, personal home, what work must be done in order for this to be started and completed?

We can relate this to building a body for a person, which is, relatively speaking, almost infinitely more complex than building a house.

First, you need a suitable piece of land for the home, and a mother's womb for a person. The land needs to be buildable and have water, sewer, electricity, natural gas, television, and telephone services available. The mother's womb has to be reasonably healthy and capable of receiving the necessary atoms and molecules as building blocks for the construction of a baby.

For the home, a *plan* is required that shows whether there is or isn't a basement or a crawl space, whether there will be one, two, or three floor levels over the foundation; the exterior size of the building; the size of the foundation walls, height, and thickness, the level of the first floor above ground; what materials to use for the foundation and how they can be properly placed, where the materials can be acquired; and who is going to do the work for building the foundation. Of course, the materials for the foundation have to be designed, manufactured, and available from another location.

For building the body of a baby, a *plan* is also required. Some of the details of the plan have to be carefully made and placed into each one of the father's millions of tiny sperm cells, and other cooperative plans have to be brilliantly and carefully made and placed into the mother's egg cells. The materials for building the sperm and egg cells have to be designed, manufactured, and available for delivery from another location away from the womb also.

For the home plan, the sizes of the rooms have to be designed: where the kitchen and bathroom(s) will be, as well as the living room, dining room, bedroom(s), closets, windows, doors, furnace, air conditioner(s), hot water heater, drains, ducts, lights, switches, plugs, chimney, stove, fridge, cabinets, plumbing, wiring, walls, roof supports, rafters, insulation, interior and exterior wall-coverings, roofing materials, stair locations, height of steps, etc.

It takes an intelligent designer to produce the plans for a house. To design a plan for a person requires *superintelligence*, far beyond that of any human group. Not only does the structure have to be suitably designed for his or her overall functions, but each one of the approximately 100 trillion complex cells in an average adult, has to be designed to live, to function, and to perform many specific living tasks reliably and consistently for anywhere from a few days to many years before God builds and installs a new replacement for it.

Each person has to choose the good foods and beverages from which God can obtain the best building-block atoms to make his or her cells. An intelligent lifestyle is also important for healthy results.

The work involved in building a nice home requires considerable knowledge and several skills, but the construction of even a huge palace is *absolutely simple* in comparison to the knowledge, skills, dexterity, precision, care, and speed required in building each and every cell of a person.

Once any home is built and finished, it requires a certain amount of care and maintenance.

However, once a baby is built and delivered into the world, it requires enormous amounts of careful work, not just to feed, clothe, wash, change diapers, teach, and other external acts, but far, far more complex and demanding is the necessary internal work of building trillions of special cells in a carefully planned and critically ordered manner to build the baby up to adult size:

1. to manufacture the food required for the baby's new cells, growth and sustenance;
2. to maintain all of the child's cells and;
3. to repair or replace all those cells that constantly need sustaining, maintaining, repairing, or replacing.

One of the favorite parts doctors examine is our red blood cells. They display a mind-boggling amount of work performed for us every second of every day just in replacing all of our roughly 20 trillion red blood cells about every 120 days. The number of required atoms that must be found in our ingested food, then sorted, selected, counted, grasped, *precisely assembled*, and delivered into our bloodstream is <u>over 4,900 quadrillion of the right atoms every second of every day</u> for every adult.[1]

Of course, *this is less than half the intelligent physical work* required to manufacture and deliver our replacement red blood cells, as, in the same second, a greater number of correct atoms must be found in the soil, air, and water in gardens and fields, etc. to be constructed into more foods for each future second's requirements for our replacement red blood cells.

A good question is, "*Why* does this superintelligent entity we call 'God' work *so hard, so reliably, and so constantly* for each one of us?

Would you agree that it must be because **He loves us** and cares immensely for each one of us all the time?.

Since He provides all of this necessary work, care, and much more to us reliably and free of charge for our entire lifetime, it is understandable why we can all rightfully say, "*In God We Can Trust.*"

In the Glossary (p. xx) we defined "God" as: "the name given by English-speaking people and governments to the superintelligent being and entity who creates and sustains all living entities....." Although we are referring to the four nations, there are many other peoples in countries where English is not the primary language, that acknowledge this same Creator God, but they have different names for Him. There are believers in China, France, Germany, India, Israel, Mexico, New Zealand, Russia,

South Africa, South Korea, and most other nations. In fact, there are people in virtually all nations of the world who acknowledge God as the Creator of life and the universe – they just use non-English names for Him.

In this book you will note that we use a capital 'H' for Him out of respect and appreciation for the enormous amount of faithful, reliable, and careful work that He performs for every person every day. In this and other textbooks to come, we will outline some of the main parts of His work for all of us.

This information is needed primarily because a deliberate exclusion of teachings about the God of our nations has occurred in most Western public schools, colleges, and universities. This exclusion seems to be based mainly on the misconception that 'evolution' as our creator is more scientific than God as Creator.

However, in fairness, many of the key, scientific details of God's amazing works for us were not previously understood or available until now.

Charles Darwin released the first edition of his book, *On the Origin of Species by Means of Natural Selection, or The Preservation of Favoured Races in the Struggle for Life* in 1859. He theorized that all life had originated from a unique happening perhaps in an ancient pond where the first living organism was formed without any intelligent help.

This organism or cell would have needed the complex ability, power, and intelligence to live, find nourishment, digest and process this nourishment to sustain its own life, eliminate waste so as not to build up toxins, produce offspring, remember its good qualities, pass these on to new cell off-spring with improvements, reproduce more cells, and over billions of years, change up to fish, animals, birds, apes, humans, etc. All this with no intelligent work or guidance.

Although this was Mr. Darwin's plagiarized idea, he mentioned the "Creator" several times. For example, in his book on *'Origins,'* Darwin says of eyesight: *"[M]ay we not believe that a living optical instrument might thus be formed as superior to one of glass, as the Works of the Creator are to those of man?"*[2]

Obviously, at this time, Darwin had great respect for the Creator and His superiority above man's abilities. Later he stated he regretted including references to "the Creator" perhaps because some of his supporters wanted God removed from his writings.

However, as noted, Darwin also outlined several ways that his theory of evolution could "absolutely break down."

We have found that for a number of the reasons, it is absolutely impossible for any living cell, organ, or living entity to be design-ed, constructed, sustained, maintained, repaired, and replaced by anything but the physical works of a superintelligent cause.

In Chapter 7 we provided seven basic principles of life indicating the need for an ultra-intelligent and caring engineering source to design, construct, and do all the work essential for all living entities, and especially us human beings.

Chapter 5 also provided a list of eighteen e*ssential intelligent physical works* required to build and maintain every living entity *which Evolution cannot do, as, by definition, it has no intelli-gence to use.*

At the time of the founding of the four nations we are addressing, not all of this science was known or available in detail for our founding fathers. However, they intuitively understood and appreciated the need for superintelligent external help with growing crops of grains, vegetables, and fruit for food, and the production of cattle for milk and meat, plus fish and fowl to eat; they knew it was reliably and faithfully supplied for the benefit of humankind by our Creator and Provider.

They called this hyperintelligent external creator and helper, 'God', just as the majority of citizens do today in these four nations. This is the same God of the Holy Bible who has been known and respected for at least several millennia of recorded history. The Holy Bible, has been the annual best-selling book in the world for centuries and has been translated into hundreds of languages and dialects.

In later chapters, which outline the role of God in the govern--ments of our nations, we will see that many of the founding fathers took time to study the wise and beneficial advice in God's "manual for operators," the Bible.

This point is made as part of the facts that help to reveal the source of the success that these four nations have enjoyed. These successes have attracted millions of immigrants from countries with other beliefs.

Today, many of our leaders pray to God for help in times of national and international distress and for His blessings for their nation and people.

When we consider all this phenomenal work that God performs for us, it is only good manners for us to thank Him. Thanksgiving Day was appropriated especially for that purpose, but it is good manners to say, "Thank you, God" often, for meals, healing, advice, prayer answers, and so on.

We may never know *all* the amazing work He performs for us.

Many people seem to believe that throwing away our moral compass is a benefit for our society, or at least for them individually. However, history and current statistics show what a destructive idea this is. (See Chapter 14.)

In 1963, Madalyn Murray (O'Hair) with some of her atheist friends, managed to convince the U.S. Supreme Court to remove prayer from public school classrooms. The concept soon spread to other nations. Since then, attempts are being made to remove all aspects of the God of our nations from public life.

Since 1963, the escalation of percentage of babies born to unwed mothers has increased, as has sexually transmitted disease, anxiety, depression, hopelessness, suicides, drug addictions, alcoholism, policing costs, ambulance costs, welfare costs, medical costs, and family breakdown, along with the trauma, heartache, and tears that go with these personal tragedies.

A major cause for these troubles lays with all who disrespect their Creator and inflict pressure to teach this disrespect. We are referring to the proponents of "Evolution-only" as the taught cause of life (inferring that God either does not exist or is not needed).

Reversing this trend will take wisdom, care, and cooperation from concerned leaders, educators, parents, and other citizens.

You can help by spreading the news that there is now a simple science called "Atomic Biology" which shows the amazing and caring works of God for everyone.

Applications for Life

1. Who can get help from the Bible? _____

_____

_____

_____

2. When is God working for us? _____

3. Does mankind have enough knowledge and intelligence to build a living cell? _____

4. Does evolution have enough ability and intelligence to build a living cell? _____

5. About how many correctly selected and counted atoms per second must be assembled just to make replacement red blood cells for an average adult? _____

References and Notes

[1] References and notes relating to the enormous work performed for each of us just in constantly replacing our red blood cells:

Pallister, C. J., *Haematology: Biomedical Science Explained,* Butterworth-Heinemann, Burlington, MA, 1999. He states that an average 70 kg adult male produces *(or has produced for him)* about 2,300,000 red blood cells every second.

Tortora, G. J., *Principles of Anatomy and Physiology,* John Wiley & Sons, New York, NY, 2008. He states that there are approximately 280,000,000 molecules of hemoglobin per red blood cell.

Perutz, Max, *Science is Not a Quiet Life: Unraveling the Atomic Mechanism of Hemoglobin,* World Scientific, Hackensack, NJ, 1997. He states that each hemoglobin molecule contains approximately 10,000 atoms.

The number of atoms required from our food and assembled into new red blood cells is approximately 2,300,000 x 280,000,000 x 10,000 = 6,440,000,000,000,000,000 (6,440 quadrillion) atoms every second of every day.

That approximate number is required for each average body for replacement red blood cells (based on a 70 kg. [154 lb.] male as average). We have conservatively used the figure of "over 4,900 quadrillion atoms per second" to include each adult in the world.

Plus, logically, in the same second an even *greater* number of atoms (for roots, leaves, etc.) from the soil, air, and water must be selected to make more food for each future second's food requirements for new red blood cell construction for each of us every second.

Again, this is in addition to the phenomenal work of constantly sustaining, maintaining, repairing, and replacing the other approximately 80 trillion cells (that require DNA) in each adult human body.

Does God deserve our appreciation? Absolutely!

[2] Darwin, Charles, *On the Origin of Species by Means of Natural Selection,* First Edition, John Murray, London, England, 1859, p. 189
available online from Darwin-online.org.uk

Chapter 10
God in the Government of the U.S.A.

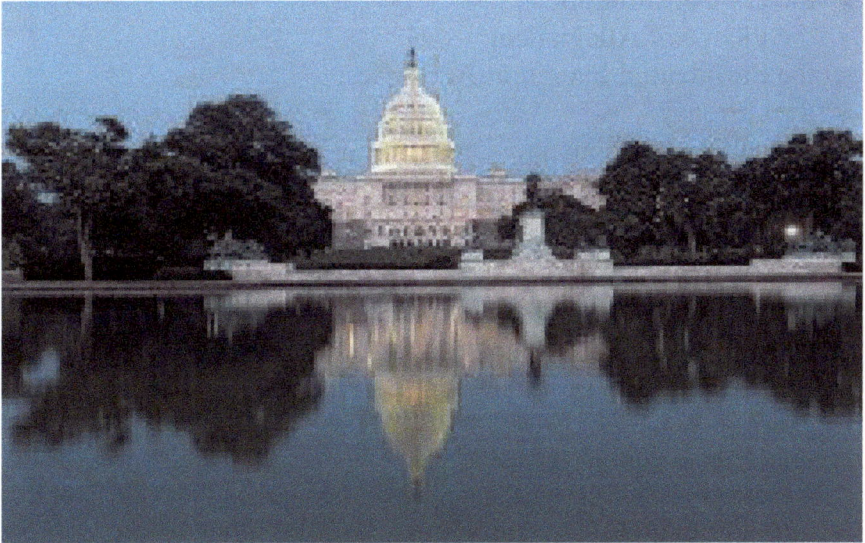

Stephen B. Goodwin/Shutterstock.com

CAPITOL HILL, U.S.A.

This chapter and the Part I science chapters show many reasons why students in the U.S.A. have the unalienable right to be taught "Why God is so highly recognized by Their Governments." He is a significant part and can provide useful knowledge for life, wisdom, encouragement, food, grace, peace, understanding, healing, and Life itself.

Our forefathers understood that God and His wise advice are integral parts of good government.

Note: Authors' emphasis by underlining.

Examples of where God has been, and is now, involved and highly recognized in the government of this nation:

- the Declaration of Independence;
- the Articles of Confederation;
- the US Constitution;
- the Pledge of Allegiance;
- the Presidential Inaugural Addresses;
- the currency;
- the national anthem and songs;
- the courts and justice systems;
- public buildings and places;
- war memorials;
- leaders' prayers and Bible studies;
- public holidays;
- majority of the citizens are believers.

As there is debate regarding the meaning of the concept of the "separation of church and state," we must stress that our Creator is *not* "the church." A church can be a building or a group of people who are Catholics, Protestants, Mormons, Jehovah's Witnesses, New Agers, Satanists, Scientologists, cults, and so on. None of them can create any living thing.

God is a highly regarded part of many churches just as He is a highly regarded part of the Government of the United States.

This high regard for God has been present in North America since before there were any formal states to be united.

The following examples of God's recognition show a few of the reasons for His importance to the nation.

Note: Author's emphasis has been added with underlining.

1. The Declaration of Independence: (Excerpts)

"In Congress, July 4, 1776. The unanimous Declaration of the thirteen United States of America: When in the Course of human events, it becomes necessary for one people to dissolve the

political bands which have connected them with another, and to assume among the powers of the earth, the separate and equal station to which the Laws of Nature and of <u>Nature's God</u> entitle them, a decent respect to the opinions of mankind requires they should declare the causes which impel them to the separation.

We hold these truths to be self-evident, that all men are <u>created</u> equal, that they are endowed by their <u>Creator</u> with certain unalienable Rights, that among these are Life, Liberty, and the pursuit of Happiness." ...

(2nd to last paragraph) *"We, therefore, the Representatives of the United States of America, in General Congress, Assembled, appealing to <u>the Supreme Judge of the world</u> for the rectitude of our intentions, do, in the Name, and by the Authority of the good People of these Colonies solemnly declare, That these United Colonies are, and of Right ought to be, Free and...Independent States;...*[1]

2. The Articles of Confederation: (Excerpts)

The thirteen Articles were officially adopted on November 15th, 1777, by representatives of the original thirteen states.

The second paragraph of Article XIII reads: *"And whereas it hath pleased the <u>Governor of the World</u> to incline the hearts of the legislatures we respectively represent in congress, to approve of, and to authorize us to ratify the said articles of confederation and perpetual union."* [2]

3. The United States Constitution: (Excerpts)

This document signed September 17, 1787, established the Government of the United States.

As a major goal of many of the early immigrants was to have freedom of religion, the U.S. Constitution helps to ensure that freedom by including the following statement in Clause 3 of Article 6: *"...no religious test shall ever be required as a qualification to any office or public trust under the United States"*[3]

Believing in God is not a legal requirement to run for high office in government. There is freedom to choose what you want to believe in, what or whom you want to have faith in, or what or whom you want to worship, if anything or anyone. It only makes good sense to choose the one that does the most for you.

4. The Pledge of Allegiance: (Excerpts)

The original version of the Pledge of Allegiance was published on September 8, 1892. It was refined periodically over the years until the present version was adopted on Flag Day, June 14th, 1954: *"I pledge allegiance to the Flag of the United States of America, and to the Republic for which it stands, <u>one nation under God</u>, indivisible, with liberty and justice for all."* [4]

5. First Presidential Inaugural Addresses:

(Excerpts are courtesy of the Lillian Goldman Law Library's Avalon Project, Yale University Law School). [5]

Note: Every President of the U.S.A. has included a request to God for His blessing on the nation, in their inaugural addresses as well as many times during their terms as President.

Only a few excerpts are shown below:

Excerpts from President George Washington's First Inaugural Address, (April 30, 1789):

"Having thus imparted to you my sentiments as they have been awakened by the occasion which brings us together, I shall take my present leave; but not without resorting once more to the benign <u>Parent of the Human Race</u> in humble supplication that, since <u>He</u> has been pleased to favor the American people with opportunities for deliberating in perfect tranquility, and dispositions for deciding with unparalleled unanimity on a form of government for the security of their union and the advancement of their happiness, so <u>His divine blessing</u> may be equally conspicuous in the enlarged views, the template consultations, and the wise measures on which the success of this Government must depend."

Excerpts from President Thomas Jefferson's First Inaugural Address, (March 4, 1801):

"Relying, then, on the patronage of your good will, I advance with obedience to the work, ready to retire from it whenever you become sensible how much better choice it is in your power to make. And may that <u>Infinite Power which rules the destinies of the universe</u> lead our councils to what is best and give them a favorable issue for your peace and prosperity."

Excerpts from President Abraham Lincoln's First Inaugural Address, (March 4, 1861):

"Why should there not be a patient confidence in the ultimate justice of the people? Is there any better or equal hope in the world? In our present differences, is either party without faith of being in the right? If the <u>Almighty Ruler of Nations, with His</u> <u>eternal truth and justice,</u> be on your side of the North, or on yours of the South, that truth and that justice will surely prevail by the judgment of this great tribunal of the American people."

.... Intelligence, patriotism, <u>Christianity, and a firm reliance on Him who has never yet forsaken this favored land</u> are still competent to adjust in the best way all our present difficulty.

You have no oath registered in heaven to destroy the Government, while I shall have the most solemn one to preserve, protect, and defend it."

Excerpts from President Franklin D. Roosevelt's Fourth Inaugural Address, (January 20, 1945):

"As I stand here today, having taken the solemn oath of office in the presence of my fellow countrymen—<u>in the presence of our God</u>—I know that it is America's purpose that we shall not fail."

In the days and in the years that are to come we shall work for a just and honorable peace, a durable peace, as today we work and fight for total victory in war."

The Almighty God has blessed our land in many ways. He has given our people stout hearts and strong arms with which to strike mighty blows for freedom and truth. He has given to our country a faith which has become the hope of all peoples in an anguished world."

So we pray to Him now for the vision to see our way clearly—to see the way that leads to a better life for ourselves and for all our fellow men—to the achievement of His will to peace on earth."

Excerpts from President Harry S. Truman's Inaugural Address, (January 20, 1949):

"The American people stand firm in the faith which has inspired this Nation from the beginning. We believe that all men have a right to equal justice under law and equal opportunity to share in the common good. We believe that all men have the right to freedom of thought and expression. We believe that all men are created equal because they are created in the image of God.

From this faith we will not be moved."

Excerpts from President Dwight D. Eisenhower's First Inaugural Address, (January 20, 1953):

"My friends, before I begin the expression of those thoughts that I deem appropriate to this moment, would you permit me the privilege of uttering a little private prayer of my own. And I ask that you bow your heads.

'Almighty God, as we stand here at this moment, my future associates in the executive

144

branch of government join me in beseeching that Thou will make full and complete our dedication to the service of the people in this throng, and their fellow citizens everywhere.

Give us, we pray, the power to discern clearly right from wrong, and allow all our words and actions to be governed thereby, and by the laws of this land. Especially we pray that our concern shall be for all the people regardless of station, race, or calling.

May cooperation be permitted and be the mutual aim of those who, under the concepts of our Constitution, hold to differing political faiths; so that all may work for the good of our beloved country and Thy glory. Amen.'

My fellow citizens: The world and we have passed the midway point of a century of continuing challenge. We sense with all our faculties that forces of good and evil are massed and armed and opposed as rarely before in history.

This fact defines the meaning of this day. We are summoned by this honored and historic ceremony to witness more than the act of one citizen swearing his oath of service, in the presence of God. We are called as a people to give testimony in the sight of the world to our faith that the future shall belong to the free.

In the swift rush of great events, we find ourselves groping to know the full sense and meaning of these times in which we live. In our quest of understanding, we beseech God's guidance.

It is because we, all of us, hold to these principles that the political changes accomplished this day do not imply turbulence, upheaval or disorder. Rather this change expresses a purpose of strengthening our dedication and devotion to the precepts of our founding documents, a conscious renewal of faith in our country and in the watchfulness of a Divine Providence.

The enemies of this faith know no god but force, no devotion but its use. They tutor men in treason. They feed upon the hunger of others. <u>Whatever defies them, they torture, especially the truth.</u>

Here, then, is joined no argument between slightly differing philosophies. This conflict strikes directly at the faith of our fathers and the lives of our sons. <u>No principle or treasure that we hold, from the spiritual knowledge of our free schools and churches</u> to the creative magic of free labor and capital, nothing lies safely beyond the reach of this struggle.

Freedom is pitted against slavery; <u>lightness against the dark.</u>

This is the hope that beckons us onward in this century of trial. This is the work that awaits us all, to be done with bravery, with charity, and <u>with prayer to Almighty God.</u>"

Excerpts from President John F. Kennedy's Inaugural Address, (January 20, 1961):

"Vice President Johnson, Mr. Speaker, Mr. Chief Justice, President Eisenhower, Vice President Nixon, President Truman, reverend clergy, fellow citizens, we observe today not a victory of party, but a celebration of freedom – symbolizing an end, as well as a beginning – signifying renewal, as well as change. For I have sworn before you and <u>Almighty God</u> the same solemn oath our forebears prescribed nearly a century and three quarters ago."

The world is very different now. For man holds in his mortal hands the power to abolish all forms of human poverty and all forms of human life. And yet the same revolutionary beliefs for which our forebears fought are still at issue around the globe – the belief that the rights of man come not from the generosity of the state, but from the hand of God."

Finally, whether you are citizens of America or citizens of the world, ask of us the same high standards of strength and sacrifice which we ask of you. With a good conscience our only sure reward, with history the final judge of our deeds, let us go forth to lead the land we love, <u>asking His blessing and His help, but knowing that here on earth God's work must truly be our own.</u>"

Excerpts from President Lyndon B. Johnson's Inaugural Address, January 20, 1965:

"My fellow countrymen, on this occasion, <u>the oath I have taken before you and before God is not mine alone, but ours together.</u> We are one nation and one people. Our fate as a nation and our future as a people rest not upon one citizen, but upon all citizens. ...

Our destiny in the midst of change will rest on the unchanged <u>character of our people, and on their faith.</u>"

We have discovered that every child who learns, every man who finds work, every sick body that is made whole – like a candle added to an altar – <u>brightens the hope of all the faithful.</u>"

<u>Let us now join reason to faith</u> and action to experience, to transform our unity of interest into a unity of purpose. For the hour and the day and the time are here to achieve progress without strife, to achieve change without hatred—not without difference of opinion, but without the deep and abiding divisions which scar the union for generations. "

"THE AMERICAN BELIEF:

Under this covenant of justice, liberty, and union we have become a nation – prosperous, great, and mighty. And we have kept our freedom. But <u>we have no promise from God that our greatness will endure.</u> We have been allowed by Him to seek greatness with the sweat of our hands and the strength of our spirit."

Our enemies have always made the same mistake. In my lifetime—in depression and in war— they have awaited our defeat. Each time, from the secret places of the American heart, came forth the <u>faith</u> they could not see or that they could not even imagine. It brought us victory. And it will again."

Excerpts from President Jimmy Carter's Inaugural Address, January 20, 1977:

<u>"Here before me is the Bible used in the inauguration of our first President, in 1789,</u> and I have just taken the oath of office on the Bible my mother gave me a few years ago, opened to a timeless admonition from the ancient prophet Micah:

<u>He hath showed thee, O man, what is good; and what doth the Lord require of thee, but to do justly, and to love mercy, and to walk humbly with thy God.'</u> (Micah 6: 8)"

<u>Ours was the first society openly to define itself in terms of both spirituality and of human liberty.</u> It is that unique self-definition which has given us an exceptional appeal, <u>but it also imposes on us a special obligation, to take on those moral duties which, when assumed, seem invariably to be in our own best interests."</u>

Let us learn together and laugh together and work together and pray together, confident that in the end we will triumph together in the right."

Within us, the people of the United States, there is evident a serious and purposeful rekindling of confidence. And I join in the hope that when my time as your President has ended, people might say this about our Nation:

> *that we had remembered the words of Micah and renewed our search for humility, mercy, and justice; that we had torn down the barriers that separated those of different race and region and religion, and where there had been mistrust, built unity, with a respect for diversity; that we had found productive work for those able to perform it; that we had strengthened the American family, which is the basis of our society; that we had ensured respect for the law, and equal treatment under the law, for the weak and the powerful, for the rich and the poor; and that we had enabled our people to be proud of their own Government once again."*

Excerpts from President Ronald Reagan's First Inaugural Address, January 20, 1981:

> *"We have every right to dream heroic dreams. Those who say that we are in a time when there are no heroes just don't know where to look. You can see heroes every day going in and out of factory gates. Others, a handful in number, produce enough food to feed all of us and then the world beyond. You meet heroes across a counter—and they are on both sides of that counter. There are entrepreneurs with faith in themselves and faith in an idea; who create new jobs, new wealth and opportunity. They are individuals and families whose taxes support the Government and whose voluntary gifts support church, charity, culture, art, and education. Their patriotism is quiet but deep.*

Their values sustain our national life.

I have used the words "they" and "their" in speaking of these heroes. I could say "you" and "your" because I am addressing the heroes of whom I speak—you, the citizens of this blessed land. Your dreams, your hopes, your goals are going to be the dreams, the hopes, and the goals of this administration, so help me God.

Above all, we must realize that no arsenal, or no weapon in the arsenals of the world, is so formidable as the will and moral courage of free men and women. It is a weapon our adversaries in today's world do not have. It is a weapon that we as Americans do have. Let that be understood by those who practice terrorism and prey upon their neighbors.

I am told that tens of thousands of prayer meetings are being held on this day, and for that I am deeply grateful. We are a nation under God, and I believe God intended for us to be free. It would be fitting and good, I think, if on each Inauguration Day in future years it should be declared a day of prayer.

Each one of those markers (in Arlington National Cemetery) *is a monument to the kinds of hero I spoke of earlier. Their lives ended in places called Belleau Wood, The Argonne, Omaha Beach, Salerno and halfway around the world on Guadalcanal, Tarawa, Pork Chop Hill, the Chosin Reservoir, and in a hundred rice paddies and jungles of a place called Vietnam.*

Under one such marker lies a young man – Martin Treptow – who left his job in a small-town barber shop in 1917 to go to France with the famed Rainbow Division. There, on the western front, he was killed trying to carry a message between battalions under heavy artillery fire.

We are told that on his body was found a diary. On the flyleaf under the heading, "My Pledge," he had written these words: "America must win this war. Therefore, I will work, I will save, I will sacrifice, I will endure, I will fight cheerfully and do my utmost, as if the issue of the whole struggle depended on me alone."

The crisis we are facing today does not require of us the kind of sacrifice that Martin Treptow and so many thousands of others were called upon to make. It does require, however, our best effort, and our willingness to believe in ourselves and to believe in our capacity to perform great deeds; to believe that <u>together, with God's help</u>, we can and will resolve the problems which now confront us.

And, after all, why shouldn't we believe that? We are Americans. <u>God bless you</u>, and thank you."

Excerpts from President George H. Bush's Inaugural Address,

January 20, 1989:

" I have just repeated word for word the oath taken by George Washington 200 years ago, and <u>the Bible on which I placed my hand is the Bible on which he placed his.</u> It is right that the memory of Washington be with us today, not only because this is our Bicentennial Inauguration, but because Washington remains the Father of our Country. And he would, I think, be gladdened by this day; for today is the concrete expression of a stunning fact: our continuity these 200 years since our government began.

We meet on democracy's front porch, a good place to talk as neighbors and as friends. For this is a day when our nation is made whole, when our differences, for a moment, are suspended.

And my first act as President is a prayer. I ask you to bow your heads:

Heavenly Father, we bow our heads and thank You for Your love. Accept our thanks for the peace that yields this day and the shared faith that makes its continuance likely. Make us strong to do Your work, willing to heed and hear Your will, and write on our hearts these words: 'Use power to help people.' For we are given power not to advance our own purposes, nor to make a great show in the world, nor a name. There is but one just use of power, and it is to serve people. Help us to remember it, Lord. Amen.

No President, no government, can teach us to remember what is best in what we are. But if the man you have chosen to lead this government can help make a difference; if he can celebrate the quieter, deeper successes that are made not of gold and silk, but of better hearts and finer souls; if he can do these things, then he must.

America is never wholly herself unless she is engaged in high moral principle.

There are few clear areas in which we as a society must rise up united and express our intolerance. The most obvious now is drugs. And when that first cocaine was smuggled in on a ship, it may as well have been a deadly bacteria, so much has it hurt the body, the soul of our country. And there is much to be done and to be said, but take my word for it: This scourge will stop.

And so, there is much to do; and tomorrow the work begins. I do not mistrust the future; I do not fear what is ahead. For our problems are large, but our heart is larger. Our challenges are great, but our will is greater. And if our flaws are endless, God's love is truly boundless.

Thank you. God bless you and God bless the United States of America."

Excerpts from President William Clinton's First Inaugural Address, January 20, 1993:

"And so, my fellow Americans, at the edge of the 21st century, let us begin with energy and hope, with faith and discipline, and let us work until our work is done. The scripture says, 'And let us not be weary in well-doing, for in due season, we shall reap, if we faint not.'"

From this joyful mountaintop of celebration, we hear a call to service in the valley. We have heard the trumpets. We have changed the guard. And now, each in our way, and <u>with God's help, we must answer the call.</u>

<u>*Thank you, and God bless you all."*</u>

Excerpts from President George W. Bush's First Inaugural Address, January 20, 2001:

"America, at its best, is a place where personal responsibility is valued and expected. Encouraging responsibility is not a search for scapegoats, it is a call to conscience. Though it requires sacrifice, it brings a deeper fulfillment. We find the fullness of life not only in options, but in commitments. We find that children and community are the commitments that set us free. Our public interest depends on private character, on civic duty and family bonds and basic fairness, on uncounted, unhonored acts of decency which give direction to our freedom. Sometimes in life we are called to do great things. But as a saint of our times has said, every day we are called to do small things with great love. The most important tasks of a democracy are done by everyone. I will live and lead by these principles, "to advance my convictions with civility, to pursue the public interest with courage, to speak for greater justice and compassion, to call for responsibility and try to live it as well." In all of these ways, I will bring the values of our history to the care of our times.

153

Americans are generous and strong and decent, not because we believe in ourselves, but because we hold beliefs beyond ourselves. When this spirit of citizenship is missing, no government program can replace it. When this spirit is present, no wrong can stand against it.

We are not this story's author, who fills time and eternity with His purpose. Yet His purpose is achieved in our duty, and our duty is fulfilled in service to one another. Never tiring, never yielding, never finishing, we renew that purpose today; to make our country more just and generous; to affirm the dignity of our lives and every life.

God bless you all, and God bless America."

Excerpts from President Barack Obama's First Inaugural Address, January 20, 2009:

"We remain a young nation, but in the words of Scripture, the time has come to set aside childish things. The time has come to reaffirm our enduring spirit; to choose our better history; to carry forward that precious gift, that noble idea, passed on from generation to generation: the God-given promise that all are equal, all are free, and all deserve a chance to pursue their full measure of happiness.

In the face of our common dangers, in this winter of our hardship, let us remember these timeless words. With hope and virtue, let us brave once more the icy currents, and endure what storms may come. Let it be said by our children's children that when we were tested we refused to let this journey end, that we did not turn back, nor did we falter; and with eyes fixed on the horizon and God's grace upon us, we carried forth that great gift of freedom and delivered it safely to future generations.

Thank you. God bless you. And God bless the United States of America."

Note: The Obama address was the last recorded by the Avalon Project at the time of this writing. All the presidential excerpts above are courtesy of the *Lillian Goldman Law Library's Avalon Project, Yale Law School.* [5]

The following two excerpts are from the *U.S. Congressional Record - Senate.*

Excerpts from President Donald Trump's Inaugural Address, *January 20, 2017:*
At the bedrock of our politics will be a total allegiance to the United States of America, and through our loyalty to our country, we will rediscover our loyalty to each other. When you open your heart to patriotism, there is no room for prejudice. The Bible tells us how good and pleasant it is when God's people live together in unity. We must speak our minds openly, debate our disagreements honestly, but always pursue solidarity. ....
Together, we will make America strong again, wealthy again, proud again, safe again, and great again.
Thank you. God bless you, and God bless America. Thank you.

Excerpts from President Joseph Biden's Inaugural Address, *January 21, 2021:*
Now, on this hallowed ground, where just a few days ago violence sought to shake the Capitol's very foundation, we come together as one nation under God, indivisible, to carry out the peaceful transfer of power as we have for more than two centuries.
Recent weeks and months have taught us a painful lesson. There is truth and there are lies, lies told for power and for profit. Each of us has a duty and a responsibility as citizens, as Americans, and especially as leaders - leaders who have pledged to honor our Constitution and protect our nation - to defend the truth and defeat the lies. .....

Let us add our own work and prayers to the unfolding story of our great Nation. If we do this, then when our days are through, our children and our children's children will say of us: They gave their best, they did their duty, they healed a broken land.

My fellow Americans, I close today where I began, with a sacred oath. <u>Before God and all of you, I give you my word.</u> I will always level with you. I will defend the Constitution. I will defend our democracy. ....

So with purpose and resolve, we turn to those tasks of our time sustained by faith, driven by conviction, and devoted to one another and the country we love with all our hearts. <u>May God bless America, and may God protect our troops.</u>

Thank you, America.

Note: The challenge for Presidents and other national leaders is to fulfill their promises and live up to a high moral standard as the role models for their nation that they are.

6. The Currency:
From the U.S. Department of the Treasury

"The Congress passed the Act of April 22, 1864. This legislation changed the composition of the one-cent coin and authorized the minting of the two-cent coin. The Mint Director was directed to develop the designs for these coins for final approval of the Secretary. <u>IN GOD WE TRUST</u> first appeared on the 1864 two-cent coin. ....

"Another Act of Congress passed on March 3, 1865. It allowed the Mint Director, with the Secretary's approval, to place the motto on all gold and silver coins that "shall admit the inscription thereon." Under the Act, the motto was placed on the gold double-eagle coin, the gold eagle coin, and the gold half-eagle coin. It was also placed on the silver dollar coin, the half-dollar coin and the quarter-dollar coin, and on the nickel three-cent coin beginning in 1866. Later, Congress passed the Coinage Act of February 12, 1873. It also said that the Secretary "may cause the motto IN GOD WE TRUST to be inscribed on such coins as shall admit of such motto." .....

"A law passed by the 84th Congress (P.L. 84-140) and approved by the President on July 30, 1956, the President approved a Joint Resolution of the 84th Congress, declaring IN GOD WE TRUST the national motto of the United States. IN GOD WE TRUST was first used on paper money in 1957, when it appeared on the one-dollar silver certificate. The first paper currency bearing the motto entered circulation on October 1, 1957. The Bureau of Engraving and Printing (BEP) was converting to the dry intaglio printing process. During this conversion, it gradually included IN GOD WE TRUST in the back design of all classes and denominations of currency." -- From the U.S. Department of the Treasury. [6]

7. The U.S. National Anthem:

"President Woodrow Wilson ordered the playing of *The Star-Spangled Banner*, at military and naval occasions in 1916, but it was not designated the national anthem by an Act of Congress until 1931.

"The words were written in 1814 by Francis Scott Key, who had been inspired by the sight of the American flag still flying over Fort McHenry after a night of heavy British bombardment. The text was immediately set to a popular melody of the time, *To Anacreon in Heaven*.

"The National Anthem consists of four verses, although on most occasions, only the first verse is sung:

Oh, say can you see by the dawn's early light
What so proudly we hailed at the twilight's last gleaming?
Whose broad stripes and bright stars thru the perilous fight,
O'er the ramparts we watched were so gallantly streaming?
And the rockets' red glare, the bombs bursting in air,
Gave proof through the night that our flag was still there.
Oh, say does that star-spangled banner yet wave
O'er the land of the free and the home of the brave?

On the shore, dimly seen through the mists of the deep,
Where the foe's haughty host in dread silence reposes,

What is that which the breeze, o'er the towering steep,
 As it fitfully blows, half conceals, half discloses?
Now it catches the gleam of the morning's first beam,
In full glory reflected now shines in the stream:
'Tis the star-spangled banner! Oh long may it wave
 O'er the land of the free and the home of the brave.

And where is that band who so dauntingly swore
That the havoc of war and the battle's confusion,
A home and a country should leave us no more!
Their blood has washed out of their foul footsteps' pollution.
No refuge could save the hireling and slave'
From the terror of flight and the gloom of the grave:
And the star-spangled banner in triumph doth wave
O'er the land of the free and the home of the brave.

Oh! thus be it ever, when freemen shall stand
Between their loved home and the war's desolation!
Blest with victory and peace, may the heav'n rescued land
Praise the Power that hath made and preserved us a nation.
Then conquer we must, when our cause it is just,
And this be our motto: 'In God is our trust.'
And the star-spangled banner in triumph shall wave
O'er the land of the free and the home of the brave." [7]

Also worth considering are the lyrics to *God Bless America*, written by Irving Berlin in 1918 and revised by him twenty years later. Like *The Star-Spangled Banner*, this tune is sung at many government functions:

God bless America,
Land that I love,
Stand beside her and guide her
Thru the night with a light from above;
From the mountains, to the prairies,
To the oceans white with foam,
God bless America,

My home, sweet home,
God bless America,
My home, sweet home.

8. U.S. Supreme Court and Justice Systems:

"When the Supreme Court opens, the Justices enter and all persons attending stand. They also stand as the Marshal of the Court chants, '*The Honorable Chief Justice and the Associate Justices of the Supreme Court of the United States. Oyez! Oyez! Oyez! All persons having business before the Honorable, the Supreme Court of the United States, are admonished to draw near and give their attention, for the Court is now sitting. <u>God save the United States and this Honorable Court!</u>*" [8]

The U.S. Supreme Court hears various arguments, and issues some one hundred and fifty annual major interpretations of the U.S. Constitution.

9. The Constitutional Oath of Office (5 USC § 3331):

Justices of the Supreme Court of the United States are required to take two oaths before they may execute the duties of their appointed office.

i. The Constitutional Oath

All federal officials must take an oath in support of the Constitution. The Constitution does not provide the wording for this oath, leaving that to the determination of Congress. From 1789 until 1861, this oath was, *"I do solemnly swear (or affirm) that I will support the Constitution of the United States."*

During the 1860s, this oath was altered several times before Congress settled on the text used today, which is set out at 5 U. S. C. § 3331. This oath is now taken by all federal employees, other than the President:

"I, _____, do solemnly swear (or affirm) that I will support and defend the Constitution of the United States against all enemies, foreign and domestic; that I will bear true faith and allegiance to the same; that I take this obligation freely, without any mental reservation or purpose of evasion; and that I will well

and faithfully discharge the duties of the office on which I am about to enter. So help me God." [9]

ii.   **The Judicial Oath**

The origin of the second oath is found in the Judiciary Act of 1789, which reads *"the justices of the Supreme Court, and the district judges, before they proceed to execute the duties of their respective offices must take a second oath or affirmation."* From 1789 to 1990, the original text used for this oath (1 Stat. 76 § 8) was:

"I, _____, do solemnly swear or affirm that I will administer justice without respect to persons, and do equal right to the poor and to the rich, and that I will faithfully and impartially discharge and perform all the duties incumbent upon me as _____, according to the best of my abilities and understanding, agreeably to the constitution and laws of the United States. So help me God."

In December 1990, the Judicial Improvements Act of 1990 replaced the phrase 'according to the best of my abilities and understanding, agreeably to the Constitution' with 'under the Constitution.' The revised Judicial Oath, found at 28 U. S. C. § 453, reads:

"I, _____, do solemnly swear (or affirm) that I will administer justice without respect to persons, and do equal right to the poor and to the rich, and that I will faithfully and impartially discharge and perform all the duties incumbent upon me as _____ under the Constitution and laws of the United States. So help me God." [10]

10. Public Buildings and Places:

The following are a few of the many places where God is referred to within, and on government buildings in Washington, D.C. For example, the Capitol Building bears many major paintings and inscriptions regarding our Creator God.

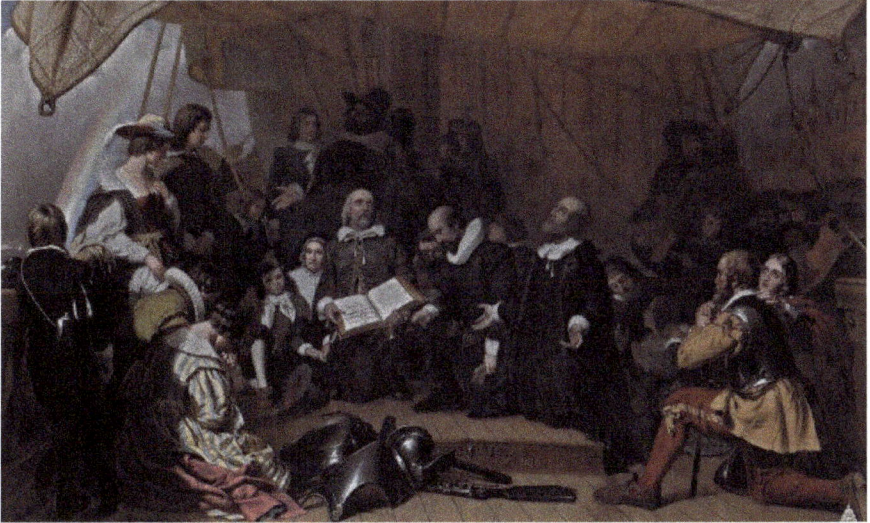

Permission by Architect of the Capitol

i. **"Embarkation of the Pilgrims"** -- *Painting by Robert W. Weir (1803 – 1889)*

This 12-foot-high by 18-foot-wide painting in the Rotunda of the Capitol Building portrays the pilgrims in 1620 on their ship *Speedwell* just before they left Holland. The words *"God with us"* were written on the sail. (You have to look closely to see the white lettering on the bottom edge of the sail in the upper-left corner). The painting shows the pilgrims with their Geneva Bible open, in prayer for success and safety in their great adventure. Their goal was to find a land where they could enjoy religious freedom.

Because of problems with the *'Speedwell,* they had to change ships in England. They booked passage on the *Mayflower* which was heading for America. This ship brought them to their new land where they established the Plymouth Colony, now known as Massachusetts.

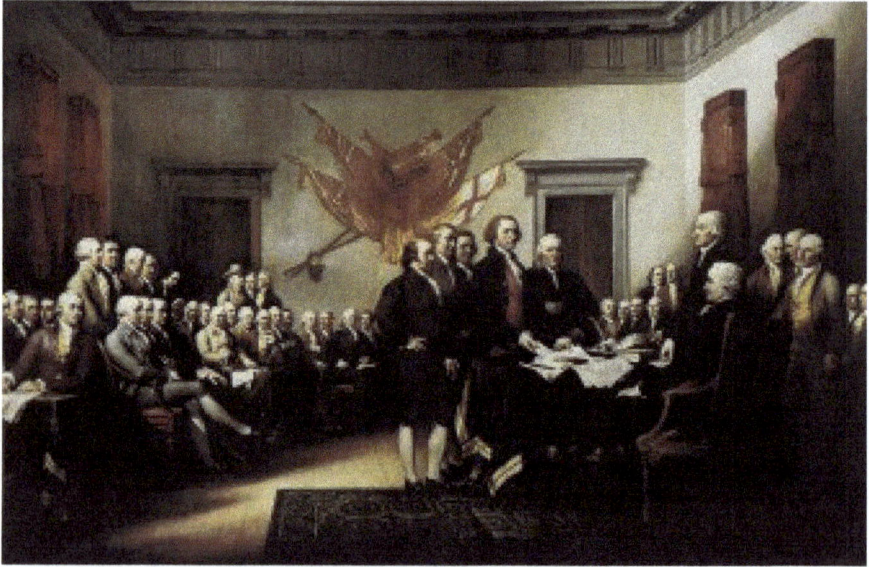

Permission by Architect of the Capitol

ii. **"Declaration of Independence, July 4, 1776"** – *Painting by John Trumbull (1756 – 1843)*

This is another 12 foot by 18 foot painting in the Rotunda of the Capitol Building. It portrays the time when the first draft of the Declaration of Independence was presented to the members of the Second Continental Congress on June 28, 1776. The document's principles remain foundational for the nation today including the words, .. *the separate and equal station to which the Laws of Nature and of Nature's God entitle them...*On July 4, 1776, the delegates from the colonies signed *The Declaration of Independence* which marked a major milestone in the development of the United States of America.

In the painting's central group, Thomas Jefferson, the principal author of the Declaration, is shown presenting the document to John Hancock, the president of the Continental Congress. Near him are other members of the committee that created the draft: John Adams, Roger Sherman, Robert Livingston, and Benjamin Franklin. The location is in what is now called Independence Hall, in Philadelphia, Pennsylvania.

iii. **Capitol Building inscriptions:**

In the Cox Corridor:
"America! <u>God shed his grace on Thee</u> and crown thy good with brotherhood from sea to shining sea!" —Katharine Lee Bates

In the House Chamber:
<u>*"In God We Trust"*</u>

In the Prayer Room:
"Annuit Coeptis" (God has favored our undertakings); and
<u>*"Preserve me, O God: for in thee do I put my trust."*</u>
—Psalm 16:1

In the Senate Chamber:
"Annuit Coeptis" (God has favored our undertakings); and <u>*"In God We Trust"*</u>

iv) **Thomas Jefferson Building inscriptions:**

Above the figure of *Religion:*
"WHAT DOES THE LORD REQUIRE OF THEE, BUT TO DO JUSTLY, AND TO LOVE MERCY, AND TO <u>WALK HUMBLY WITH THY GOD.</u>"
Quoted from the Holy Bible, Micah 6:8

Above the figure of *Science:*
<u>"THE HEAVENS DECLARE THE GLORY OF GOD;</u>
AND THE FIRMAMENT SHEWETH HIS HANDIWORK".
Quoted from the Holy Bible, Psalms 19:1" [11]

11. War Memorials:

From the records of the American Battle Monuments Commission, the following are a few examples of the U.S. war memorials that contain the name of God or Biblical references:

i. **The Arlington National Cemetery**, Arlington, Virginia: On its Chaplains Monument, dedicated to military clergy who fell in the First World War, are inscribed the words "<u>TO THE</u>

163

<u>GLORY OF GOD</u> AND THE MEMORY OF THE CHAPLAINS WHO DIED IN SERVICES OF THEIR COUNTRY" and <u>"MAY GOD GRANT PEACE TO THEM AND TO THE NATION THEY SERVED SO WELL"</u>.

ii. **The National Memorial Arch**, Valley Forge, Pennsylvania: This monument includes the words "...THIS VALLEY IN THE SHADOW OF THAT DEATH...", which is based on Psalm 23, verse 4.

iii. **The Liberty War Memorial**, Kansas City, Missouri: It was built to honor the fallen American soldiers of the First World War. Its inscription includes the statement "THEIR BODIES RETURN TO DUST", which is a reference to Genesis, 3:19.

iv. **The American Military Cemetery**, Manila, Philippines: It contains the largest number of war graves of U.S. military dead (17,202) who were casualties of the Second World War. There are also names of 36,286 military personnel missing in action inscribed in special walls. The memorial bears the inscription: <u>"GRANT UNTO THEM O LORD - ETERNAL REST WHO SLEEP IN UNKNOWN GRAVES."</u>

v. **The Cambridge American Cemetery**, Cambridge, England: This is the resting place of fallen Americans from the First and Second World Wars. It contains a memorial with the inscription "HERE LIES IN HONORED GLORY <u>A COMRADE IN ARMS KNOWN BUT TO GOD."</u>

vi. **The Normandy American Cemetery**, Normandy, France: This is a final resting place for American military personnel fallen in both the First and Second World Wars. A memorial there bears the inscriptions "HERE RESTS IN HONORED GLORY <u>A COMRADE IN ARMS KNOWN TO GOD</u>" and <u>"MINE EYES HAVE SEEN THE GLORY OF THE COMING OF THE LORD."</u>

vii. **The Brookwood American Cemetery and Memorial**, Brookwood, England: This location honors Americans who lost their lives in the First World War. An inscription there reads "HERE RESTS IN HONORED GLORY <u>AN AMERICAN SOLDIER KNOWN BUT TO GOD…</u>"

viii. **The Florence American Cemetery and Memorial** near Florence, Italy: Dedicated to U.S. military personnel lost in the Second World War, it has a panel which bears the inscription "…<u>O GOD WHO ART THE AUTHOR OF PEACE . . .</u>"

God made every one of us and I am sure it hurts Him when we kill each other. However, He does fully understand defense against evil.

12. Leaders' Prayers:

In times of regional, national, or international distress, it is noticeable to hear in person and through media, presidents provide prayers for the hurting.

Other political leaders, such as governors and mayors, have prayed for God's help in times of suffering, pain, and grief. We see and hear this repeatedly in the media, whether it is part of disaster relief, or in the aftermath of shootings, or other violent acts. Many of these leaders have prayed for God's guidance in their work of governing. Unfortunately, not all leaders do this.

13. Leaders' Bible Studies:

On Capitol Hill in Washington, DC, there are Bible studies, such as the Congressional Prayer Caucus, for those elected members who wish to attend.

14. U.S. Public Holidays Intended for Honoring God:

The major public holidays in the U.S. intended for honoring God are Good Friday, Easter Sunday, Thanksgiving Day, and Christmas.

i. **Good Friday:** This major public holiday is celebrated the Friday before Easter Sunday. The week leading up to Good Friday is sometimes celebrated as Holy Week. It commem-orates the crucifixion of Jesus Christ as His sacrificial payment of the penalty for our spiritual sins. *Spiritual redemption is a gift we only have to accept in order to receive.*

ii. **Easter Sunday:** is a day to celebrate the resurrection of Jesus Christ after his death. It is the "Third Day" on which Jesus rose from the dead, as described in the New Testament. Easter Monday is also a holiday, but it does not have the significance of the immediately preceding days.

iii. **Thanksgiving Day:** President George Washington issued a Proclamation in 1789 to declare a time for official thanks to God. It read as follows:

"By the President of the United States of America

– A Proclamation

Whereas it is the duty of all Nations to acknowl-edge the providence of Almighty God, to obey his will, to be grateful for his benefits, and humbly to implore his protection and favor—and Whereas both Houses of Congress have by their Joint Committee requested me to recommend to the People of the United States a day of public thanksgiving and prayer to be observed by acknowledging with grateful hearts the many signal favors of Almighty God, especially by affording them an opportunity peaceably to establish a form of government for their safety and happiness. . .

Given under my hand at the City of New York the third day of October in the year of our Lord 1789, Geo. Washington." [12]

Days of thanksgiving and praise to God for His provisions of foods and other blessings have been celebrated since the days of the pilgrims and other early colonists.

In the U.S., Thanksgiving Day is now celebrated on the fourth Thursday of November each year. One of this major holiday's traditions is to have a special meal with family and/or friends, and give thanks to God for His harvest foods and other blessings.

iv. **Christmas**: This is an annual commemoration of the birth of Jesus Christ, the central figure in the Godhead or Holy Trinity of Father, Son, and Holy Spirit. Christmas is a widely observed holiday celebrated on December 25th by multi-millions of people around the world.

The above examples are just a small sampling of God's involvement with the government of the United States. There is much more regarding His reference, respect, and influence federally, as well as all His involvement in state and county affairs. It is reasonable, logical, and important that citizens, including students, be taught who the God of their nation *is*, as well as what he does for each one of us every day. Now there is the new science of "Atomic Biology" to verify God as our Creator.

15. Current Believers in God in the U.S.A.:

RELIGION ACCORDING TO GALLUP POLL, JULY 20, 2023
BY **MEGAN BRENAN**

HIGHLIGHTS
-   **74% believe in God, 69% angels, 67% heaven, 59% hell, 58% the devil;**
-   **Nearly three in 10 do not believe in hell or the devil;**
-   **Belief greatest among frequent churchgoers, Protestants, Republicans.**

WASHINGTON, D.C. -- The percentages of Americans who believe in each of five religious entities -- God, angels, heaven, hell and the devil -- have edged downward by three to five percentage points since 2016. Still, majorities believe in each, ranging from a high of 74% believing in God to lows of 59% for hell and 58% for the devil. About two-thirds each believe in angels (69%) and heaven (67%).

Gallup has used this framework to measure belief in these spiritual entities five times since 2001, and the May 1-24, 2023, poll finds that each is at its lowest point. Compared with 2001, belief in God and heaven is down the most (16 points each), while belief in hell has fallen 12 points, and the devil and angels are down 10 points each.

Bottom Line

Gallup has consistently documented sharp declines in <u>church attendance</u>, <u>confidence in organized religion</u> and <u>religious identification</u> in recent years. Americans' beliefs regarding God, angels, heaven, hell and the devil have also fallen by double digits since 2001. Still, U.S. adults' belief in each entity remains at the majority level, and regular churchgoers, Protestants and Republicans, in particular, remain largely resolute in their beliefs.

Earlier in this book we provided many solid, scientific reasons for this belief.

Applications for Life

1. Would you agree that God is a highly recognized part of the Government of the United States? _____

2. In your opinion, what about God makes Him important to the Government? _____

_____

_____

_____

3. What do you think the reasons were for establishing Thanksgiving Day? _____

_____

_____

4. What is the National Motto of the U.S.A. and where is it shown most often? _____

_____

5. Have most or all of the Presidents recognized God? _____

6. Do you remember hearing a President or a government representative praying to God in times of a national or international distress; who and about what problem? _____

_____

_____

7. In these Declaration of Independence words, please fill in the blanks: *We hold these truths to be self-evident, that all men are* _____, *that they are endowed by*

_____ *with certain unalienable Rights, that among these are Life, Liberty, and the pursuit of Happiness."* ...

8. In the Pledge of Allegiance, the words include *"...one nation under* _____ ."

9. In the great song, "_____ *Bless America,*" do you think He will continue to do that if we do not show our appreciation for Him and all he work He provides for each of us every second of every day?

_____

10. Do you think that all citizens, both young and old, can help to make America a wiser and better (more Godly) nation again, meaning more caring, less violent, more moral, and more thankful, and how? _____

_____

_____

_____

References and Notes:

[1] "Declaration of Independence," *The Charters of Freedom,* The U.S. National Archives and Records Administration, College Park, MD, http://www.archives.gov/exhibits/charters/declaration.html; accessed March 1, 2014.

[2] "Transcript of Articles of Confederation (1777)," *Our Documents,* http:/www.ourdocuments.gov/doc.php?doc=3&page=transcript; accessed March 1, 2014.

[3] "Transcript of Constitution of the US (1787)," *Our Documents,* http://www.ourdocuments.gov/doc.php?doc=9&page=transcript; accessed March 1, 2014.

[4] "U.S. Pledge of Allegiance to the Flag," http://www.publications.usa.gov/epublications/ourflag/pledge. Html; accessed March 3, 2014.

[5] Courtesy of the Lillian Goldman Law Library's Avalon Project, Yale University Law School, http://avalon.law.yale.edu/subject_menus/inaug.asp; accessed March 3, 2014.

[6] "History of 'In God We Trust,'" U.S. Department of the Treasury, http://www.treasury.gov/about/education/Pages/ingod-we-trust.aspx; accessed March 3, 2014.

[7] "The U.S. National Anthem," U.S. Army Music, http://www.music.army.mil/music/nationalanthem/; accessed March 3, 2014.

[8] "The Court and Its Procedures," Supreme Court of the United States, Washington, D.C., http://www.supremecourt.gov/about/procedures.aspx; accessed March 5, 2014.

[9 & 10] "Text for the Oaths of Offices for Supreme Court Judges," Office of the Curator, Supreme Court of the United States, Washington, DC, http://www.supremecourt.gov/about/oath/textoftheoathsofoffice2009.pdf; accessed March 4, 2014.

[11] "The Thomas Jefferson Building," *On These Walls: Inscriptions and Quotations in the Buildings of the Library of Congress,* U.S. Library of Congress, Washington, DC, http://www.loc.gov/loc/walls/jeffl.html; accessed June 16, 2014.

[12] "Thanksgiving in North America: From Local Harvests to National Holiday," Smithsonian, Washington, D.C., http://www.si.edu/Encyclopedia_SI/nmah/thanks.htm; accessed March 5, 2014.

Chapter 11

God in the Government of the U.K.

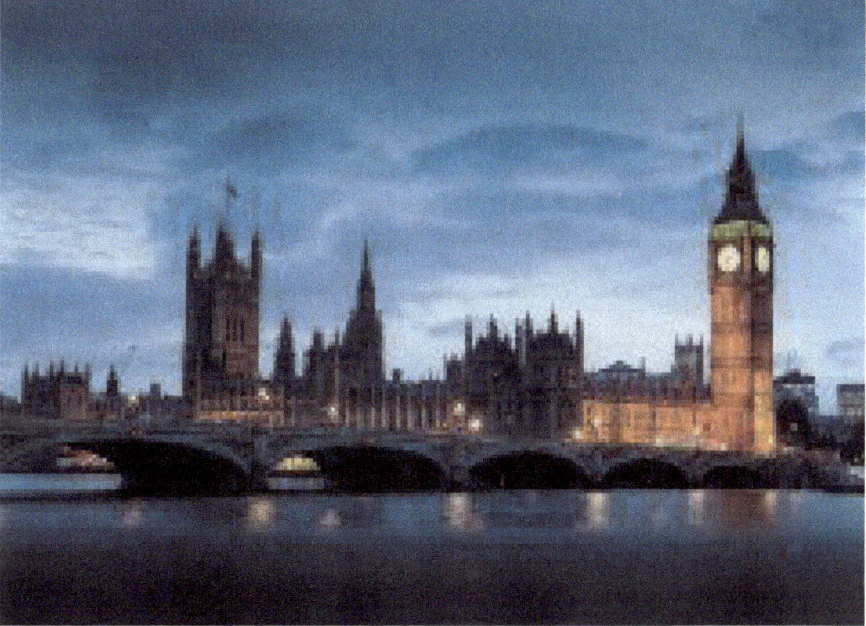

Alice-photo/Shutterstock.com

PALACE OF WESTMINISTER - U.K. PARLIAMENT

So, Who IS This 'God' of Our Nation? This chapter and the science chapters show many reasons why students in the U.K. have the right to be taught "Why God is so highly recognized by Their Government." He is a significant part and can provide wisdom, hope, encouragement, food, grace, peace, understanding, knowledge, and Life itself.

Our forefathers understood that God and His wise advice are integral parts of good government.

Shown in this chapter are a few of the areas where God in the U.K. Government has been acknowledged in:

- the monarchy;
- the courts and justice systems;
- parliamentary oaths and sovereignty;
- the constitution;
- the national anthem;
- the Prime Ministers' speeches;
- the currency;
- national buildings and places;
- government publications;
- war memorials;
- parliamentary prayers;
- national holidays;
- believers.

The following examples of God's recognition show His importance to the nation:

(The following quotes from U.K. National Archives contain public sector information licensed under the Open Government Licence v2.0. This does not infer an endorsement of its use herein).

Note: Author emphasis by underlining. "Misspellings are actually correct Early Modern (Shakesperean) English and/or British spellings of the words.

1. God's Involvement with some of the United Kingdom's Monarchs:

i. The Coronation Oath of King William and Queen Mary

"I: ...The *Coronation Oath Act, 1688*, when employed at Coronations, uses the <u>King James Bible.</u>

"II: Oath hereafter mentioned to be adminstered, by the <u>Archbishop of Canterbury,</u> ...

"May it please Your Majesties That the Oath herein Mentioned and hereafter Expressed shall and may be Adminstred to <u>their most Excellent Majestyes King William and Queene</u>

Mary whome God <u>long preserve</u> at the time of Their Coronation in the presence of all Persons that shall be then and there present at the Solemnizeing thereof by the <u>Archbishop of Canterbury or the Archbishop of Yorke</u> or either of them or any other Bishop of this Realme whome the King's Majesty shall thereunto appoint and who shall be hereby thereunto respectively Authorized which Oath followeth and shall be Administred in this Manner That is to say,

"III: Form of Oath and Adminstration thereof. E+W

"The <u>Arch Bishop or Bishop</u> shall say,

"Will You solemnely Promise and Sweare to Governe the People of this Kingdome of England and the Dominions thereto belonging according to the Statutes in Parlyament Agreed on and the Laws and Customs of the same?   "The King and Queene shall say, "I solemnly Promise soe to doe.

<u>"Arch Bishop or Bishop,</u>

"Will You to Your power cause Law and Justice in Mercy to be Executed in all Your Judgements.

"King and Queene,

"I will.

<u>"Arch Bishop or Bishop.</u>

<u>"Will You to the utmost of Your power Maintaine the Laws of God the true Profession of the Gospell</u> and the Protestant Reformed Religion Established by Law? And will You Preserve unto the Bishops and Clergy of this Realme and to the Churches committed to their Charge all such Rights and Priviledges as by Law doe or shall appertaine unto them or any of them.

"King and Queene.

"All this I Promise to doe.

"After this the King and Queene laying His and Her Hand upon the <u>Holy Gospells,</u> shall say,

"King and Queene

"The things which I have here before promised I will performe and Keepe <u>Soe help me God.</u>

"Then the King and Queene shall kisse the Booke.

"IV: Oath to be adminstered to all future Kings and Queens.

"And the said Oath shall be in like manner Adminstred to every King or Queene who shall Succeede to the Imperiall Crowne of this Realme at their respective Coronations by one of the Archbishops or Bishops of this Realme of England for the time being to be thereunto appointed by such King or Queene respectively and in the Presence of all Persons that shall be Attending Assisting or otherwise present at such their respective Coronations Any Law Statute or Usage to the contrary notwithstanding." [1]

ii. **The Coronation Oath from the Coronation of Charles III,** May 6, 2023 .

The <u>Archbishop of Canterbury</u> conducted this oath, administering it in the form of questions:

"*Archbishop*: Will you solemnly promise and swear to govern the Peoples of the United Kingdom of Great Britain and Northern Ireland, your other Realms and the Territories to any of them belonging or pertaining, according to their respective laws and customs?

"*King*: I solemnly promise so to do.

"*Archbishop*: Will you to your power cause Law and Justice, in Mercy, to be executed in all your judgements?

"*King*: I will.

"*Archbishop*: Will you to the utmost of your power maintain the Laws of God and the true profession of the Gospel? Will you to the utmost of your power maintain in the United Kingdom the Protestant Reformed Religion established by law? Will you maintain and preserve inviolably the settlement of the Church of England, and the doctrine, worship, discipline, and government thereof, as by law established in England? And will you preserve unto the Bishops and Clergy of England, and to the Churches there committed to their charge, all such rights and privileges, as by law do or shall appertain to them or any of them.

"*King*: All this I promise to do.

"Then the King places his hand on the Bible and says, "The things which I have here before promised, I will perform and keep. <u>So help me God.</u>

" Then the king kisses the Bible.

"*Archbishop:* Your Majesty, are you willing to make, sub-scribe, and declare to the statutory Accession Declaration Oath?
"*King:* I am willing.

"I, Charles, do solemnly and sincerely in the presence of God profess, testify, and declare that I am a faithful Protestant, and that I will, according to the true intent of the enactments which secure the Protestant succession to the Throne, uphold and maintain the said enactments to the best of my powers according to law.

"The King signs copies of the Oaths, by the Lord Chamberlain, whilst the choir sings, 'Prevent us, O Lord, in all our doings with thy most gracious favour, and further us with thy continual help; that in all our works begun, continued, and ended in thee, we may glorify thy holy name, and finally by thy mercy obtain everlasting life; through Jesus Christ. Amen'.

"*William Byrd (c 1540-1623) The Book of Common Prayer 1549.*

"*The King kneels before the altar and says,'* God of compassion and mercy whose Son was sent not to be served but to serve, give grace that I may find in thy service perfect freedom and in that freedom, knowledge of thy truth. Grant that I may be a blessing to all thy children, of every faith and belief, that together we may discover the ways of gentleness and be led into the paths of peace; through Jesus Christ our Lord. Amen.'
The King returns to the Chair of Estate and sits. " [2]

2. Judicial Oaths

When judges are sworn in they take two oaths/affirmations. The first is the oath of allegiance and the second, the judicial oath; these are collectively referred to as the judicial oath.

i. Oath of Allegiance

"I, _____ , do swear by Almighty God that I will be faithful and bear true allegiance to His Majesty King Charles the Third, his heirs and successors, according to law." [3]

ii. **Judicial Oath**

"I, _____ , do swear <u>by Almighty God</u> that I will well and truly serve our Sovereign King Charles the Third in the office of _____ , and I will do right to all manner of people after the laws and usages of this realm, without fear or favour, affection or ill will." [4]

3. Parliamentary Oaths

"In the House of Commons, after election, an MP must swear an Oath of Allegiance before taking his or her seat. Members who object to swearing an oath may make a Solemn Affirmation instead.

"In the House of Lords the Oath of Allegiance must be taken, or Solemn Affirmation made, by every Lord on introduction and at the beginning of every new Parliament. This must be done before he or she can sit and vote in the House of Lords. "While holding a copy of the New Testament (or, in the case of a Jew or Muslim, the Old Testament or the Koran) a Member swears: "I, _____ , swear <u>by Almighty God</u> that I will be faithful and bear true allegiance to His Majesty King Charles, his heirs and successors, according to law. So help me God."

"The text of the affirmation is: – "I, ... , do solemnly, sincerely and truly declare and affirm that I will be faithful and bear true allegiance to His Majesty King Charles, her heirs and successors according to law". [5]

"In the United Kingdom, a significant part of the formal State Opening of Parliament is a Speech from the Throne. This is currently made by His Majesty, King Charles III. The Speech outlines the main bills to be introduced in the session of parliament and concludes with the statement, "My Lords and Members of the House of Commons, <u>I pray that the blessing of Almighty God</u> may rest upon your counsels." [6]

4. Parliamentary Sovereignty and the U.K. Constitution

"Parliamentary sovereignty is a principle of the U.K. constitution. It makes Parliament the supreme legal authority in the U.K., which can create or end any law. Generally, the courts cannot overrule its legislation and no Parliament can pass laws that future Parliaments cannot change. Parliamentary sovereignty is the most important part of the U.K. constitution.

"People often refer to the U.K. having an 'unwritten constitution' but that's not strictly true. It may not exist in a single text, like in the U.S.A. or Germany, but large parts of it are written down, much of it in the laws passed in Parliament – known as statute law.

"Therefore, the U.K. constitution is often described as 'partly written and wholly uncodified'. (Uncodified means that the U.K. does not have a single, written constitution.) ...." [7]

Therefore, the various statutes that recognize God, are part of the constitution.

5. National Anthem
GOD SAVE THE KING

God save our gracious King,
Long live our noble King,
God save the king!
Send him victorious ,
Happy and glorious,
Long to reign over us;
God save the King!
Thy choicest gifts in store
On him be pleased to pour;
Long may he reign;
May he defend our laws,
And ever give us cause
To sing with heart and voice,
God save the King! [8]

6. Prime Ministers' Speeches Wherein God was Recognized

Many British Prime Ministers including Churchill, Thatcher, Brown, Cameron, and others have made statements regarding Britain's reliance on God's help with the survival, success, and well-being of the United Kingdom.

7. Currency

Today, most U.K. coins recognize God through the inscription "DEI GRATIA REGINA" or an abbreviation, "DEI GRA REG," or "D. G. REG." These all mean, "By the Grace of God, King" (or Queen). Another term that appears on the currency is "FIDEI DEFENSOR," "FID DEF," or "F.D." which all mean "Defender of the Faith."

This is another recognition of God by the Government of the United Kingdom (aka 'His Majesty's Government').

8. National Buildings and Places

Within the United Kingdom many public buildings bear inscriptions or artistic works that acknowledge God. (We address war memorials separately, later in this chapter.)

The following are examples of a few inscriptions in Westminster Abbey:

i. On a processional cross: "Nation shall not lift up sword against nation, neither shall they learn war anymore." From the Bible, Isaiah 2:4. [9]

ii. On an Abbey bell: "Christie Audi Nos" which translated means "Christ Hear Us" [10]

iii In the south aisle of the nave, on a monument to Carola Morland, second wife of Sir Samuel Morland, a Gentleman of the Privy Chamber, "Blessed be thou of the Lord, my honoured wife! Thy memory shall be a blessing, O virtuous woman." [11]

iv. Below each dial of "Big Ben" on the Elizabeth Tower, Palace of Westminster, the following inscription carved in stone: "Domine Salvam fac Reginam nostrum Victoriam primam" which means "O Lord, save our Queen Victoria the First". [12]

9. God in Government Publications

Take as an example the "Companion to the Standing Orders and Guide to the Proceedings of the House of Lords."

The "Appendix K" in this official document contains choices of Biblical verses that can be read to the House of Lords, as well as the option of six possible prayers to be read for opening each sitting of the House. [13]

10. War Memorials

The **U.K. National Inventory of War Memorials (UKNIWM)** was founded in 1989 to build a comprehensive record of every war memorial (roughly 100,000) in the United Kingdom, (including England, Scotland, Wales, and Northern Ireland), plus the Isle of Man and the Channel Islands. The name has since been changed to the Imperial War Museums War Memorials Archive. The following are just a few of the war memorials that bear inscriptions acknowledging God, besides honouring the heroes who gave their lives defending the people of their nation:

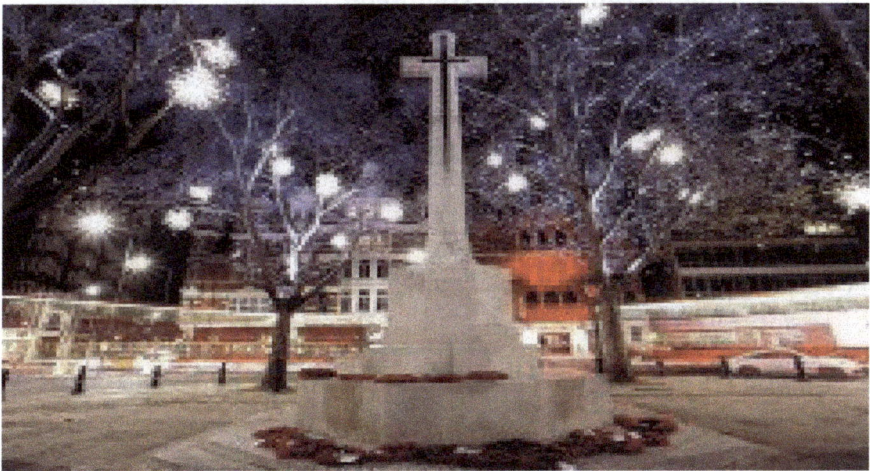

Bikeworldtravel/Shutterstock.com

WAR MEMORIAL AT SLOANE SQUARE, LONDON

i. The West Hartlepool War Memorial, Hartlepool, Cleveland, England. Also known as the Victory Square War Memorial or the Victory Square Cenotaph. It commemorates those who died in the First and Second World Wars and includes the inscription: "…Thine O Lord Is The Victory."

ii. First World War Memorials:

These include Ayton War Memorial, in Ayton, Berwickshire; the Earlston War Memorial, in Earlston, Berwickshire; the Gordon War Memorial, in Gordon, Berwickshire; and the

Whitsome War Memorial, in Whitsome, Berwickshire. All are inscribed "To the glory of God ..." The Whitsome War Memorial includes a second plaque, honoring those who fell in the Second World War, which is also inscribed "To the glory of God ..."

iii. **The Ford and Etal War Memorial,** Ford, Northumberland: It consists of two marble tablets: the first one is dedicated to the memory of those who fell in the First World War and reads "Grant them, O Lord, eternal rest." The second tablet, immediately below it, is dedicated to those who died in the Second World War.

iv. **The Anglo-French War Memorial,** Thiepval, Picardie, France: It commemorates those who lost their lives in the Battle of the Somme or in the First World War. The British headstones are inscribed with the phrase: "A Soldier of the Great War/Known to God."

v. **The Scottish National War Memorial**, Edinburgh, Scotland: includes the inscription "Thanksgiving and Praise to God" and "To the Glory of God."

vi. **The National Monument to the Women of World War II,** Whitehall, London, England. It contains a frieze with an inscription that concludes with the words "Glory be to God on high and on earth peace." [14]

11. Prayers in Parliament

Both the House of Commons and the House of Lords open their sessions with prayers. These are read by the chaplain in the Commons and by the senior bishop in the House of Lords.

"The form of the main prayer (in Commons) is as follows: "*Lord, the God of righteousness and truth*, grant to our King and his government, to Members of Parliament and all in positions of responsibility, the guidance of your Spirit. May they never lead the nation wrongly through love of power, desire to please, or unworthy ideals but laying aside all private interests and prejudices keep in mind their responsibility to seek to improve the condition of all mankind; *so may your kingdom come and your name be hallowed. Amen.* ^" [15]

The senior bishop in the House of Lords can consult the "Companion to the Standing Orders" for a *choice of prayers* to read. (See Point 9 "God in Government Publications" earlier in this chapter, p. 181).

12. U.K. National Holidays in God's Honour

i.   **Good Friday** is the Friday before Easter Sunday. The week leading up to Good Friday is sometimes celebrated as Holy Week. Good Friday is a major religious holiday. *It commemorates the crucifixion of Jesus Christ* as His sacrificial payment of the penalty for our spiritual sins. Spiritual redemption is a gift we only have to accept in order to receive.

ii. **Easter Sunday** (holiday taken on Easter Monday) *is a day to celebrate the resurrection of Jesus Christ* after his death.   It is the "third day" of His sacrificial time and is the day He arose from His dead state, as described in the New Testament and historically established.

iii.   **Harvest Festival of Thanksgiving** *is a celebration to thank our Creator and Provider for the harvest of food grown on the land in the current year.* It is also about giving thanks for all the good gifts in our lives such as family, friends, pets, flowers, and other created blessings.

iv. **Christmas** is *an annual commemoration of the birth of Jesus Christ, the central figure in the Godhead or Holy Trinity of Father, Son, and Holy Spirit.* Christmas is a widely observed holiday, generally celebrated on December 25 by multi-millions of people around the world.

This is just a small sampling of God's involvement with the national government of the United Kingdom. There is much more regarding His recognition, respect, and influence nationally, as well as all His involvement at the county level. *It is reasonable, logical, and important that all U.K. citizens, including students, be taught who this God of their nation is and what he does for each of us every second of every day.*

Religious Composition of England and Wales

The 2021 data show that the largest changes since 2011 were for those describing their religion as "Christian" and those reporting "No religion." (Note: 'mil' = million).

Religious composition, 2011 and 2021, England and Wales:

	2011	2021
Buddhist	0.4% (249,000)	0.5%(273,000)
Christian	59.3% (33.3 mil.)	46.2% (27.5 mil.)
Hindu	1.5% ((818,000)	1.7% (1.0 mil.)
Jewish	0.5% (265,000)	0.5% (271,000)
Muslim	4.9% (2.7 mil.)	6.5% (3.9 mil.)
Sikh	0.8% (423,000)	0.9% (524,000)
Other religion	0.4% (241,000)	0.6% (348,000)
No religion	25.2% (14.1 mil.)	37.2% (22.2 mil.)
Not answered	7.1% (4.0mil.)	6.0% (3.6 mil.)

Of those who wrote-in a non-religious group to "Any other religion", the largest numbers were:
- Agnostic (32,000)
- Atheist (14,000)
- Humanist (10,000)

Source: Office for National Statistics – Census 2021

In the 2011 Census in **Scotland**, of 5,295,000 covered, 2,850,000 (about 54%) indicated that they were Christian, while 2,309,000 indicated they either had no religion or did not answer the question regarding their religion. [17]

In the 2022 Census, the population rose to 5,436,000. The increase in people with no religion in Scotland coincided with a decrease in people who said they belong to the Church of Scotland. In 2022, 20.4% responded 'Church of Scotland', down from 32.4% in 2011 and from 42.4% in 2001. This is a fall of

610,100 people since 2011, and over 1 million since 2001. However 'Church of Scotland' remained the largest group among those who said they had a religion.

The next largest religious groups were 'Roman Catholic' (13.3%), 'Other Christian' (5.1%) and 'Muslim' (2.2%). These groups saw smaller changes since the last census than 'Church of Scotland'. The number of people who described themselves as Roman Catholic decreased by 117,700 since 2011, whilst the number in the Other Christian category decreased by 12,000. The number of people who described themselves as Muslim increased by 43,100 over the same period. [18]

In the 2021 Census in **Northern Ireland**, 1,844,500 were enumerated, out of a total population of 1,903,100. Of these, 1,475,800 (about 80.0%) claimed to be Christian, 23,400 (about 1.3%) other religion, while 345,100 (about 18.7%) claimed no religion or did not answer the religion question. [19]

Applications for Life

1. Would you agree that God is a highly recognized part of the government of the United Kingdom? _____

2. What is it about God that makes Him important to the Government in your opinion?

_____

_____

_____

3. What do you think the reasons were for establishing the Harvest Festival? _____

_____

_____

4. If you were God and you were working constantly to make vegetables and fruit and meat for everyone to eat every day, then you made and maintained their cells using the atoms from the food,

but many people never said, "Thank you, God" even once, what would you think?

_____

_____

5. What is the National Anthem of the U.K. and what are some of the occasions when it is sung? _____

_____

6. Have most or all of the Prime Ministers recognized God? ___

_____

7. Do you remember hearing a Prime Minister or a government representative praying to God in times of a national or international distress; who and about what problem? _____

_____

8. At the State Opening of Parliament in the U.K., what are the words of the last sentence that the Queen (or King) says after reading the outline of the main bills to be introduced in that session of parliament? _____

_____

_____

9. In the Oath of Allegiance, the words are: "I, _(name)___ , do swear by _____ that I will be faithful and bear true allegiance to His Majesty King Charles the Third, his heirs and successors, according to law." _____

_____

10. Do you think that all citizens, both young and old, can help to make the U.K. a wiser and better (more Godly) nation again, meaning more caring, less violent, more moral, and more thankful, and how?

_____

References and Notes:

[1] "Coronation Oath Act, 1688," The National Archives, Government of the United Kingdom,
   http://www.legislation.gov.uk/aep/WillandMar/1/6, Richmond, Surrey, England, accessed March 6, 2014.

[2] "Coronation Oath, 6 May, 2023," The full text of the Coronation Oath of King Charles III,
   https://www.countrylife.co.uk/coronation, accessed February 22, 2024.

[3 & 4] "Oaths," Courts and Tribunal Judiciary, London, England,
   http://www.judiciary.gov.uk/about-the-judiciary/oaths/, accessed March 6, 2014.

[5] "Oath of Allegiance," U.K. Parliament, London, England,
   http://www.parliament.uk/site-information/glossary/oath-ofallegiance/, accessed March 8, 2014.

[6] "Oath of Allegiance," U.K. Parliament, London, England,
   http://www.publications.parliament.uk/search/results/?q=Oath+of+allegiance, accessed May 2, 2014.

[7] "Parliamentary Sovereignty," U.K. Parliament, London, England,
   http://www.parliament.uk/about/how/sovereignty/, accessed May 2, 2014.

[8] "National Anthem," The British Monarchy,
   http://www.royal.gov.uk/MonarchUK/Symbols/NationalAnthem.aspx, accessed March 7, 2014.

[9] "Processional Crosses", Westminster Abbey, London, England,
   http://www.westminster-abbey.org/worship/processionalcrosses,accessed July 24, 2014.

[10] "Abbey Bells," Westminster Abbey, London, England, http://www.westminster-abbey.org/our-history/abbey-bells, accessed July 24, 2014.

[11] "Carola Morland," Westminster Abbey, London, England, http://www.westminster-abbey.org/our-history/people/carolamorland, accessed July 24, 2014.

[12] "Big Ben: The Clock Dials," U.K. Parliament, London, England, http://www.parliament.uk/about/livingheritage/building/palace/big-ben/building-clock-tower/clockdials/, accessed July 25, 2014.

[13] "Appendix J: Prayers for the Parliament," *Companion to the Standing Orders and Guide to the Proceedings of the House of Lords,* 2013 edition, U.K. Parliament Publications, http://www.publications.parliament.uk/pa/ld/ldcomp/compso2013/Part3_14.htm, accessed August 12, 2014.

[14] War Memorials Archive, Imperial War Museum, London, England, http://www.ukniwm.org.uk and various links; accessed June 13, 2014.

[15] "Prayers," U.K. Parliament, London, England, http://www.parliament.uk/about/how/business/prayers, accessed June 14, 2014.

[16] "Religion by measures," Nomis, Durham England, http://www.nomisweb.co.uk/census/2011/KS209EW/view/2092957703?cols=measures, accessed July 31, 2014.

[17] "Summary: Religious Group Demographics, 2011," The Scottish Government, Edinburgh, Scotland, http://www.scotland.gov.uk/Topics/People/Equality/Equalities/DataGrid/Religion/relPopMig, accessed July 31, 2014.

[18] https://www.scotlandscensus.gov.uk/2022-results/scotland-s-census-2022-ethnic-group-national-identity-language-and-religion/, accessed May 21, 2024

[19] https://www.nisra.gov.uk/system/files/statistics/census-2021-population-and-household-estimates-for-northern-ireland-statistical-bulletin-24-may-2022.pdf:, accessed May 21, 2024.

Chapter 12

God in the Government of Australia

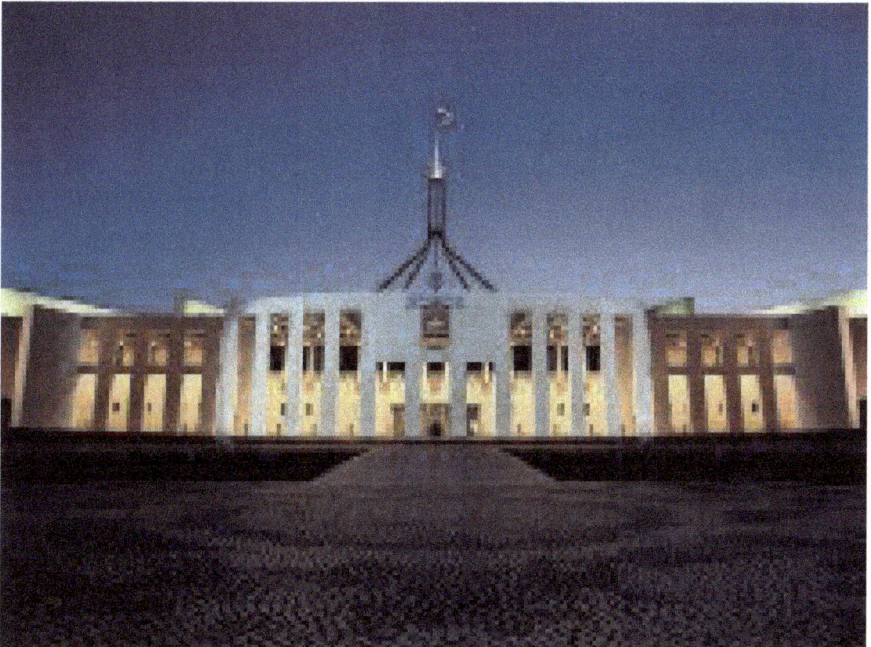

Dan Breckwoldt/Shutterstock.com

PARLIAMENT HOUSE, CANBERRA

So, Who IS This 'God' of Our Nation? This chapter and the science chapters show many reasons why students in Australia have the unalienable right to be taught "Why God is a highly recognized part of their Government." He can provide His wisdom, hope, encouragement, grace, under-standing, and useful knowledge for their life enjoyment. He also produces all their grown foods and their Life itself..

Our forefathers understood that God and His wise advice are integral parts of good government.

189

Note: Author's emphasis added by underlining.

European Discovery and Settlement of Australia

Two adventurous, European navigators, Christopher Columbus in 1492 and Ferdinand Magellan in 1519, sailed west across the Atlantic Ocean in search of a shorter route to India for trading. Both believed that God guided them and protected them on these dangerous journeys of discovery. Columbus discovered the Americas and Magellan was the first navigator whose ship and surviving crew were the first to sail around the world. Unfortunately, Magellan was killed in the Philippines. Neither adventurer found Australia but they showed a way for others.

The western side of Australia was discovered by sailors such as William Dampier. Although he was a confirmed rogue, Dampier, stated in the preface to his book, *A Voyage to New Holland, an English Voyage of Discovery to the South Seas in 1699*, "But this Satisfaction I am sure of having, that the Things themselves in the Discovery of which I have been employed, are most worthy of our diligentest (sic) Search and Inquiry; being the various and wonderful Works of God in different Parts of the World." [1]

However, it was not until 1770 that Captain James Cook discovered the east coast of Australia and claimed it for Great Britain.

Matthew Flinders, who had the honour of naming Australia, was the first to circumnavigate the continent in 1802/1803 with this goal, "... to make so accurate an investigation of the shores of Terra Australis that ...with the blessing of God, nothing of importance would be left for future discoverers upon any part of these extensive coasts." [2]

European Settlement

"Governor Arthur Phillip arrived from England with the first fleet in 1788 to settle Australia with soldiers and criminals who could no longer be transported to North America because of American Independence.

His instructions were to *"enforce a due observance of religion and good order among the inhabitants and take such steps for the due celebration of public worship as circumstances would permit. In the first draft of these instructions he was to grant full liberty of conscience, and the free exercise of all modes of religious worship not prohibited by law, provided his charges were content with a quiet and peaceable enjoyment of the same, not giving offence or scandal to government; he was to cause the laws against blasphemy, profaneness, adultery, fornication, polygamy, incest, profanation of the Lord's Day, swearing and drunkenness to be rigorously executed. He was not to admit to the office of justice of the peace any person whose ill-fame or conversation might occasion scandal; he was to take care that the Book of Common Prayer as by law established be read each Sunday and Holy Day, and that the Blessed Sacrament be administered according to the rites of the Church of England. Because of the great disproportion of female to male convicts, he was to take on board at any of the islands any women who might be disposed to come, taking care not to make use of any compulsive measures or fallacious pretences. He was to emancipate from their servitude any of the convicts who should, from their good conduct and a disposition to industry, be deserving of favour, and to grant them land, victual them for twelve months and equip them with tools, grain, and such cattle, sheep and hogs as might be proper, and could be spared. As the military officers and others might be disposed to cultivate the land, he was to afford them every encouragement."* [3]

Other nations could have settled Australia but mostly their beliefs prevented them from doing so: Hindus prevented sea voyages and contact with foreigners; a revolution in China in 1433 ended the voyages of navigator Cheng Ho; before the 1400s, Muslim sailors believed the southland was Dedjdal or the kingdom of Antichrist; and European expansion had begun in the East Indies and Pacific ending the expansion of Islam.

Early Leadership in Australia

Most of the colonies' early leadership came from the evangelical Christian community, mainly chaplains. Governors such as Hunter, Macquarie, and Brisbane, and a number of officials such as Judge Advocates Wylde and Ellis Bent, the editor of Australia's first newspaper, were strongly committed to Christian views, as were the schoolteachers.

Governor Macquarie was always trying to improve the moral and religious well-being of the colony, hoping that those in his care would become good Christians. He personally promoted the *British and Foreign Bible Society and the Sunday School Movement.* He also encouraged other Christian groups such as the Auxiliary Bible Society and spoke at the Inaugural meeting. Macquarie particularly encouraged Christian education starting a number of schools under the supervision of the government chaplains so that by 1817 the most common discussion in the pages of the Sydney Gazette was on the merits of Bible reading. *James Stephen, the Permanent Under Secretary of the Colonial Office, believed that God was going to sovereignly use Australia as a Christian nation.* He thought that it should be governed by Biblical principles and encouraged Christian families to settle here. Hence, he was influential in the choice of *Christian leaders in the colonizing of the country.*

Australia's modern education system was pioneered by the chaplains and remained overtly Christian up to the 1880s. After that, it became more secular with the Anglican Church aligning with independent denominations in an unsuccessful attempt to stop the influence of Catholicism.

In 2011, the federal government increased funding for chaplaincy in public schools. That same year, attempts to remove the date designations "BC" (Before Christ) and "AD" (Anno Domini, Latin for "in the year of our Lord") from the national history curriculum were defeated.

South Australia's Godly Beginnings and the Aspirations of Its Founders

For many years South Australia's capital, Adelaide, was known as the Holy City, but today it is called the City of Churches. In its formative years, Adelaide did not have enough churches for all of its parishioners.

During Adelaide's first eight years there were more preachers and places of worship than in the first decade of settled life in New England in the United States. From the time of South Australia's settlement in 1836 to 1915 more children attended Sunday school than attended regular school. In one of the first schools opened by Richard Angas, the sole textbook was the Bible. Angas distributed millions of gospel tracts in his lifetime.

Prayer and Meditation

Sir George Grey, a South Australian governor, shared with James Stephen in the Colonial Office, the view that "prayer and meditation on *God's Holy Word*...were the inexhaustible, unfathomable source of all pure consolation and spiritual strength." [4]

Later, Grey was instrumental in the founding of New Zealand. New Zealand recently celebrated the bicentenary of the gospel arriving on its shores on Christmas Day, 1814, by the Reverend Samuel Marsden.

Godly Elements in Australia's Foundation

1. Law and Parliament

Australia's common law has been based on the Christian faith, exemplified by the statue of Jesus that occupied the central place above the Royal Courts of Justice in London, and many statements made by scholars. One Chief Justice declared: "Christianity is parcel of the Common Law of England and therefore to be protected by it. So whatever strikes at the very root of Christianity tends manifestly to the dissolution of civil government." Australia's oldest parliament in New South Wales (NSW) governed most of Australia and many of the South Pacific islands including New Zealand. Today it still opens with this prayer: *"Almighty God, we ask for your blessing upon this Parliament. Direct and prosper our deliberations to the true welfare of Australia and the people of New South Wales. Amen."* Parliament of New South Wales Standing Orders 39. [5]

A similar prayer is said in our Federal Parliament by the President, who, upon taking the chair each day, reads the following prayer: *"Almighty God, we humbly beseech Thee to vouchsafe Thy special blessing upon this Parliament, and that Thou wouldst be pleased to direct and prosper the work of Thy servants to the advancement of Thy glory, and to the true welfare of the people of Australia.*

"Our Father, which art in Heaven, Hallowed be Thy name. Thy kingdom come. Thy will be done in earth, as it is in Heaven. Give us this day our daily bread. And forgive us our trespasses, as we forgive them that trespass against us. And lead us not into temptation; but deliver us from evil: For thine is the kingdom, and the power, and the glory, for ever and ever. Amen." [6]

Alfred Deakin, the man mainly responsible for the passage of the Australian Constitution through the English House of Commons, repeatedly prayed over this significant document.

During this time, just prior to the turn of the century, Christians were coming together to discuss the federation movement (the alignment of separate states into one country). Many wanted to see God recognized as the ruler of the nation. Hence, it was carried unanimously in the Constitutional Convention that the preamble to Australia's Constitution should include the phrase, *"...humbly relying on the blessing of Almighty God."* Deakin was delighted with this outcome. (See next item, Our 1901 Commonwealth Constitution).

Deakin became Australia's second prime minister, after Edmund Barton, whose Presbyterian minister, Dr. Robert Steele, had inspired him to enter politics. The fourth prime minister, Sir George Reid, was also inspired to enter politics through Dr. Steele's influence. Deakin, who was born in Australia, was nurtured in his faith by his mother. It was Deakin who seconded the motion put forth by "Father of Federation" Sir Henry Parkes, for the proposed Federation of the Australian States.

Deakin kept a spiritual diary and from 1884 to 1913 wrote a *Boke of Praer and Praes* which contained nearly four hundred prayers. They mainly related to major decisions in his public life, revealing his utter dependence on God.

In the concluding words of his book *The Federal Story,* Deakin remarks that the Federation and the Australian Constitution were "providential" and were secured only "by a series of miracles."

In his notes in 1905 Deakin remarks, *"Sufficient to say that the religion of Jesus Christ is the life of the present, the light of the future and the hope of the world."* Many years later he stated: *"A life, the life of Christ, that is the one thing needful – the only revelation required is there... we have but to live it."* [7]

A Christian statesman, Deakin was the first Attorney General of the Commonwealth, and as such, founder of the High Court of Australia. He served three times as prime minister when a considerable amount of the Commonwealth's initial legislation started. As prime minister he founded the Arbitration Court, and the Australian Navy, as well as choosing Canberra as the nation's capital.

On June 3rd, 1898 a polling day was held in N.S.W., Victoria, and Tasmania to vote on creating a federation. By midnight Deakin knew that Victoria had approved the bill by an overwhelming majority, that Tasmania had done likewise, but that the majority in New South Wales had not reached the minimum number required for the adoption of the Bill. Hence, Deakin prayed, *"Father of Nations, receive our psalm of thanksgiving. Enable us to pursue the cause of unity in spite of the obstacles which at present appear to beset our path elsewhere. Guide us to appeal to that which is best and purest so as to make its development and mastery sure under our forms of government. Aid us to purify ourselves by our labours for the general weal and to invoke spiritual and moral principles so as to link us with our brethren on the highest plane to which we can at present attain. God preserve this people and grant its leaders unselfish fidelity and courage to face all trials for the sake of brotherhood. Thy blessing has rested upon us here yesterday and we pray that it may be the means of creating and fostering throughout all Australia a Christ-like citizenship."* [8]

2. The 1901 Commonwealth Constitution

The Preamble to the Australian Constitution states: *"Whereas the people of New South Wales, Victoria, South Australia, Queensland, and Tasmania, <u>humbly relying on the blessing of Almighty God,</u> have agreed to unite in one indissoluble Federal Commonwealth under the Crown of the United Kingdom of Great Britain and Ireland, and under the Constitution hereby established..."* These words are quoted from the Commonwealth of Australia Constitution Act, 1900. [9]

This preamble was in response to numerous signed petitions from people from every colony represented in the Federal Convention. This acknowledgement of the sovereignty of God was approved unanimously.

It is unlikely that Federation of the States would have been approved if the preamble had not included reference to Almighty God, as alluded to by Mr. Lyne (N.S.W.) in the debate. Some members of the constitutional convention had reservations, but with the inclusion of section 116, this was resolved and the "recognition insertion" was carried unanimously. Section 116 states:

"The Commonwealth shall not make any law for establishing any religion, or for imposing any religious observance, or for prohibiting the free exercise of any religion, and no religious test shall be required as a qualification for any office or public trust under the Commonwealth." These words are quoted from the Commonwealth of Australia Constitution Act, 1900. [10]

3. Monarchy

<u>Our Constitutional Christian Monarchy expresses the Lordship of Christ when the King or Queen is presented with the Bible:</u> *"...to keep your Majesty ever mindful of the law and the Gospel of God as the rule for the whole of life and government of Christian Princes, we present you with this Book, the most valuable thing this world affords. Here is wisdom; this is the royal law; these are the lively oracles of God."* [11]

When the royal orb is delivered to the King or Queen, the coronation service states: *"Receive this Orb set under the cross and remember that the whole world is subject to the power and empire of Christ our Redeemer."* [12]

4. The Flag

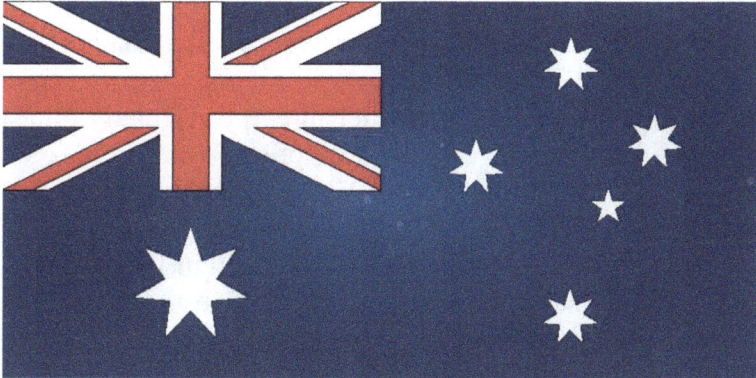

Artgraphixel.com/Shutterstock.com

The Australian flag bears four Christian crosses. It incorporates the Southern Cross, which God has placed in the Southern Hemisphere, along with the crosses of St Andrew (white stripes on blue), St Patrick (back red on white), and St. George (front red on white).

5. Australian Days of Prayer

On June 11, 1738, John Wesley, a Christian theologian and Anglican cleric, blew the first trumpet call of the great evangelical revival. This was to have a deep and lasting effect on Britain and those in succeeding generations, prompting some to immigrate to Australian shores. Today, Wesley and his brother Charles are credited with founding the Methodist Church movement.

Fifty years after the arrival of the first fleet, the NSW Governor, George Gipps – a Christian – proclaimed Sunday, November 2, 1838, a national day of fasting and humility because of severe drought. Within two days, heavy rains began to fall.

Almost six decades later on September 11, 1895, a day of prayer was again called in similar circumstances. Three weeks later a day of thanksgiving was proclaimed to thank God for the breaking of the drought.

Even the editorial in the April 14, 1897, edition of the Sydney Morning Herald stated: *"No Christian could in conscience vote for a Federation Bill that did not recognise God!"*

The first Sunday in the twentieth century was proclaimed Commonwealth Sunday and Christians were called to pray for the nation. During the 1940s the Second World War began to take its horrific toll and Australia was under threat, particularly after the bombing of Darwin. Several days of prayer were held; one of these was called by King George VI, to be held throughout the British Commonwealth.

Australia's biggest prayer meeting was held in 1988 during the country's bicentenary celebrations. Thirty-five thousand people surrounded the New Parliament House in Canberra, the nation's capital, representing triple the number who attended the official opening.

In 2004, the Governor-General of the Commonwealth of Australia, His Excellency Major General Michael Jeffery, fulfilled the desire of many Christians in Australia and launched a National Day of Thanksgiving. It was celebrated for the first time on May 29, 2004. In 2011, the inaugural National Day of Prayer and Fasting was held and in 2012 the inaugural National Christian Heritage Sunday took place on the first Sunday in February commemorating the first sermon on Australian soil on the 3rd day of February, 1788.

6. Opening of the Australian Parliament May 9, 1901 – A Christian Service

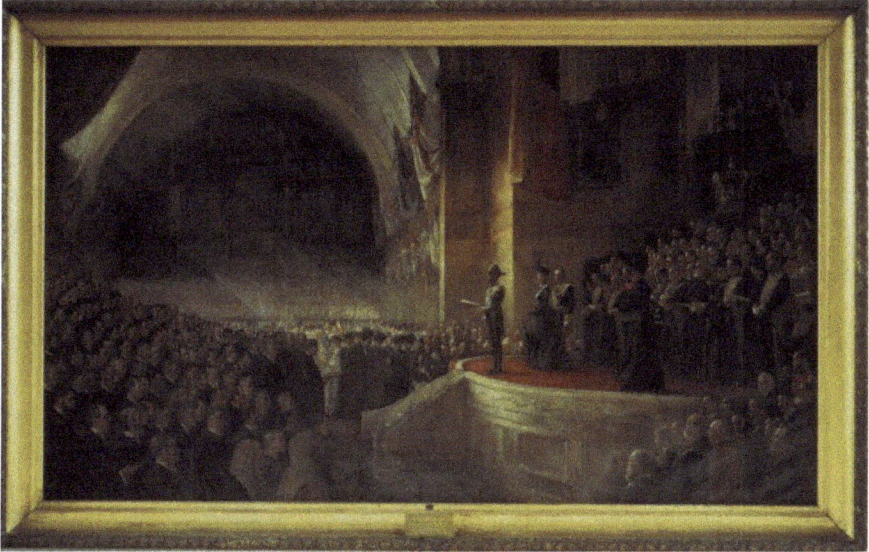

Royal Collection Trust / © Her Majesty Queen Elizabeth II, 2014
This painting is on permanent loan to the parliament of Australia
from the British Royal Collection. [13]

The opening of Parliament of the Commonwealth included the singing of Psalm 100, accompanied by an orchestra with His Excellency the Right Honourable the Earl of Hopetoun, a Member of His Majesty's Most Honourable Privy Council; Knight of the Most Ancient and Most Noble Order of the Thistle, Knight Grand Cross of the Most Distinguished Order of Saint Michael and Saint George, Knight Grand Cross of the Royal Victorian Order, Governor-General and Commander-in-Chief of the Common-wealth of Australia, reading the following prayers:

"O Lord, our heavenly Father, high and mighty, King of kings, Lord of lords, the only Ruler of princes, who dost from Thy throne behold all the dwellers upon earth, most heartily we beseech Thee with Thy favour to behold our most gracious Sovereign Lord King Edward, and so replenish him with the grace of Thy Holy Spirit that he may always incline to Thy will and walk in Thy way. Endue

him plenteously with heavenly gifts, grant him in health and wealth long to live, strengthen him that he may vanquish and overcome all his enemies; and finally, after this life he may attain everlasting joy and felicity, <u>through Jesus Christ our Lord.</u> – Amen. "Almighty God, the fountain of all goodness, we humbly beseech Thee to bless our gracious Queen Alexandra, George Duke of Cornwall and York, the Duchess of Cornwall and York, and all the Royal Family; endue them with Thy Holy Spirit; enrich them with Thy heavenly grace; prosper them with all happiness; and <u>bring them to Thine everlasting Kingdom, through Jesus Christ our Lord.</u> – Amen.

"Almighty God, we humbly beseech Thee to regard with Thy merciful favour the people of this land, now united in one Commonwealth. We pray for Thy servants the Governor-General, the Governors of the States, and all who are or who shall be associated with them in the administration of their several offices. "We pray Thee at this time to vouchsafe Thy special blessing upon the Federal Parliament now assembling for their first session, and that Thou wouldst be pleased to direct and prosper all their consultations to the advancement of Thy glory and to the true welfare of the people of Australia, through Jesus Christ our Lord, who has taught us when we pray to say:

"Our Father, which art in heaven, hallowed be Thy name. Thy kingdom come. Thy will be done in earth as it is in heaven. Give us this day our daily bread. And forgive us our trespasses, as we forgive them that trespass against us. And lead us not into temptation; but deliver us from evil; for Thine is the kingdom, and the power, and the glory, forever and ever. – Amen.

"The grace of our Lord Jesus Christ, and the love of God, and the fellowship of the Holy Ghost, be with us all, evermore. – Amen." [14]

The Australian Parliamentary Christian Fellowship conducts an annual Australian National Prayer Breakfast, under the oversight of the Parliamentary Chaplain in the Great Hall, in Parliament House, Canberra. It is attended by many dignitaries from Australia and overseas.

7. Currency

i. The Australian twenty-dollar note features Rev. John Flynn (1880-1951), who founded the Flying Doctor Service and the Australian Inland Mission. His Presbyterian ministers or Patrol Padres were known as the boundary riders of the bush, who rode camels to complete their mission work in central Australia. Flynn was responsible for using the pedal-wireless, a radio transmitter-receiver, to establish communication throughout inland Australia. This provided a new mantle of support and protection over the region, which was the size of Western Europe.

On the bottom-right-hand corner of the note is an image of one of the five camels that Flynn purchased in 1913 for his Patrol Padres.

ii. A picture of Pastor David Unaipon appears on the fifty-dollar note. An aboriginal, Unaipon was a writer, inventor, and pastor. A church is visible on the bottom left corner of the bill.

iii. An image of Caroline Chisholm (1808–1877) appeared on the five-dollar note for more than twenty years until 1992 when polymer notes were introduced. Married in the Church of England, she converted to her husband's religion of Catholicism. She first arrived in New South Wales in 1838 then worked to establish better conditions, including suitable employment and accommodation, for young migrant women. Her work expanded to include making families' passage to Australia easier. What Australia needed most, in her view, were "good and virtuous women." In six years, she settled eleven thousand people as servants and farmers in NSW.

8. Swearing on the Bible in Court and Parliament

In courts, the Christian oath states: *"The evidence you shall give to the Court [and jury sworn] shall be the truth, the whole truth, and nothing but the truth, <u>so help you God</u>. Say 'I swear.' The witness then says, 'I Swear.'"*

Most people still swear on the Bible rather than make an affirmation, according to a criminal defense lawyer in Adelaide.

Most parliamentarians, prime ministers, and cabinet ministers are sworn in using the Bible. The Governor-General invites these officials to stand in their place and take the Bible in their right hand. The oath is read with the reply *"I do. So help me God!"* Prayers in local governments often appear in written form or are read by a clergy member.

9. Our Charitable Institutions

Thankfully, most of today's major Australian charitable and welfare agencies, such as the Salvation Army, Anglicare, Wesley Centre in Sydney and St. Vincent de Paul Society, continue as Christian institutions. Christian churches, more so than in England and the U.S., have been responsible for the development of social services.

10. Public Holiday – ANZAC Day on April 25th

Public holidays in Australia include Easter, Christmas, Australia Day, and the Queen's birthday. Throughout Australia and New Zealand, ANZAC (Australia New Zealand Army Corp) Day remembers our fallen soldiers in memorial services in virtually every town and suburb. They invariably are solemn Christian services such as the one led by a local pastor, held in Orange, N.S.W. in 2012, shown in the following photo. His public address included many Biblical references and concluded with a benediction.

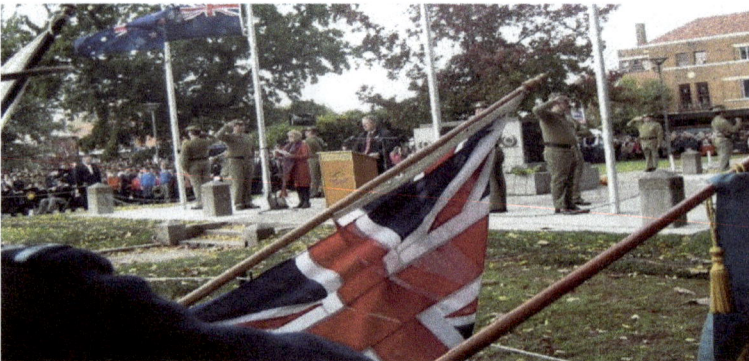

Courtesy of Graham McLennan

202

11. ANZACS and Israel

The Australian and New Zealand armed forces commonly known as ANZACS have served in both the First and Second World Wars, as well as other theatres of war. One of the group's major achievements was the Australian Light Horse charge at Beersheba, on October 31, 1917, with eight hundred men on horseback. God was using one of the newest nations in the world to take Jerusalem from the Turks and Germans. This liberated Jerusalem from four hundred years of rule under the Turkish Ottoman Empire. Neither the military genius of Napoleon, nor the British Army with fifty thousand British Infantry who had fought bravely, had been successful in this challenge.

On the day of the Beersheba charge, the British government drafted the Balfour Declaration, which later became the foundation for the recognition of the State of Israel.

At every ANZAC service, the *Recessional Hymn*, written by the English poet and author, Rudyard Kipling in 1897, is sung:

God of our fathers, known of old
Lord of our far-flung battle line
Beneath Whose awful Hand we hold
Dominion over palm and pine
Lord God of Hosts, be with us yet,
Lest we forget, lest we forget. [15]

This hymn has become even more famous as the source of the oft-quoted phrase *"Lest we forget,"* used in ANZAC Day ceremonies.

Conclusion

We can see that Australia's discovery, settlement and growth can easily be explained in terms of God's intentions for this nation. He has used His men and women to lead in so many areas of development that even the most humanistic historian would have difficulty explaining away the mass of evidence at which this chapter only hints.

If the past is misinterpreted then so is the significance of the future. It is important that we don't continue to be deceived by the secularization process which denies the sovereignty of God in our history, past and present.

For further understanding of Australia's Christian heritage, please refer to the website of the Australian Christian History Research Institute (www.chr.org.au).

Current Believers in God in Australia:

The following excerpts were taken from the Australian Bureau of Statistics:

2071.0 - Census of Population and Housing: Reflecting Australia - Stories from the Census, 2016

POPULATION AT CENSUS TIME (2016) 23,401,892

LATEST ISSUE Released at 11:30 AM (CANBERRA TIME) 28/06/2017

RELIGION IN AUSTRALIA, 2016

INTRODUCTION

The religious fabric of the world is changing. Increased migration has dispersed religious ideas and practices throughout the world. Changes in social attitudes have also influenced how people see themselves and their relationship with religion.

The Australian population is no different. In the 1911 Census of Population and Housing, 96% of Australians reported Christianity as their religion. Today we have more diversity in religions and denominations, as well as an increasing number of people reporting that they do not have a religion.

MAJOR RELIGIOUS AFFILIATIONS IN 2016 and 2021 [16]

Reflecting the historical influence of European migration to Australia, Christianity was the most common religion reported in the 2016 Census (52%), with Catholics the largest group (23% of the population). Other religions make up a much smaller proportion of the population (8.2%), with the most commonly reported being Islam (2.6%), closely followed by Buddhism (2.4%). Nearly a third (30%) of Australians reported that they had no religion in 2016.

Compared with the 2011 Census, the proportion of the population with a Christian affiliation decreased from 61% to 52% in 2016. Conversely, the proportion of the population with a religion other than Christianity increased from 7.2% in 2011 to 8.2% in 2016. The proportion reporting to have no religion also increased from 22% in 2011 to 30% in 2016 (over an additional 2 million persons).

RELIGIOUS AFFILIATIONS: 2021 - Population 25,422,788

In 2021, more people opted to answer the Census religion question than in 2016. In 2021, the number of people who answered the religion question was 93.1% of the population, an increase from 90.9% in 2016.

In 2021 the most common religions were:

- Christianity (43.9%)
- No religion (38.9%)
- Islam (3.2%)
- Hinduism (2.7%)
- Buddhism (2.4%)

Decline in Christian Affiliation

The number of people affiliated with Christianity in Australia decreased from 12.2 million (52.1%) in 2016 to 11.1 million (43.9%) in 2021. This decrease occurred across most ages, with the largest decrease for young adults (18-25 years).

Decrease in Christian Denominations – 2016 to 2021

Christian denomination	Decrease
Anglican	-604,900
Catholic	-215,900
Uniting Church	-196,900
Presbyterian and Reformed	-111,800
Lutheran	- 28,200
Salvation Army	- 13,600
Pentecostal	- 4,700
Latter-day Saints	- 3,800
Churches of Christ	- 3,700
Other Christian	- 2,900

Source: Religious affiliation (RELP).

Applications for Life

1. Would you agree that God is a highly recognized part of the Government of Australia? _____

2. What is it about God that makes Him important to the Government in your opinion? _____

_____

_____

_____

_____

3. What do you think the reasons were for establishing Christmas and Easter as national holidays? _____

_____

_____

4.   What are the three descriptions of God in the traditional ANZAC hymn? _____

_____

_____

5. Who were three of the early Governors of Australia who were believers in God? _____

_____

6. Do you remember hearing a Prime Minister or a government representative praying to God in times of a national or international distress; who and about what problem? _____

_____

_____

7. What is the first sentence of the prayer read at the opening of federal parliament each day? _____

_____

_____

_____

_____

_____

8. In the preamble to the Australian Constitution, who are the states relying on for blessings? _____

9. Do you think that all citizens, both young and old, can help to make Australia a wiser and better (more Godly) nation again,

meaning more caring, less violent, more moral, and more thankful, and how? _____

_____

_____

References and Notes:

1   Dampier, W., *A Voyage to New Holland, an English Voyage of Discovery to the South Seas in 1699,* facsimile edition, 1981, accessible at Project Gutenberg, Salt Lake City, UT, www.gutenberg.org/files/15675/15675-h/15675-h.htm, accessed August 12, 2014.

2   Scott, E., *The Life of Matthew Flinders,* Angus & Robertson, Sydney, AU, 1914, p.272.

3   Clark, C.M.H.., *A History of Australia Vol.1,* University Press, Melbourne, AU, 1962, p.80.

4   Clark, C.M.H., *A History of Australia Vol.3: The Beginning of an Australian Civilization, 1824-1851,* University Press, Melbourne, AU, 1973, p.40.

5   *Standing Orders, Legislative Assembly, Parliament of New South Wales,* p. 12, Parliament of New South Wales, Sydney, http://www.parliament.nsw.gov.au/Prod/la/precdent.nsf/0/0D8 13F110566E803CA2572A500059E36/$file/standing%20order s%202010.pdf, accessed August 12, 2014.

6   "Prayer and acknowledgement of country," *Chapter 8: Sittings, quorum, and adjournment of the Senate, Powers, Practice, and Procedure, Parliament of Australia, Canberra, AU,* http://www.aph.gov.au/About_Parliament/Senate/Powers_practice_ n_procedures/aso/so050, accessed March 7, 2014.

7   La Nauze, J., *Alfred Deakin, A Biography,* Angus & Robertson, Sydney, AU, 1979, pp.70, 79.

8   McLennan, G., *Understanding Our Christian Heritage,* vol. 2,
    prayer 223, Christian History Research Institute, Orange, NSW,
    Australia, 1989, p. 80.

9   "Commonwealth of Australia, Constitution Act," Powers,
    Practice, and Procedure, Parliament of Australia, Canberra, AU,
    www.aph.gov.au/About_Parliament/Senate/Powers_practice_n
    _procedures/Constitution/preamble; accessed March 8, 2014.

10 "Commonwealth of Australia, Constitution Act," *Chapter V:
    The States,* Powers, Practice, and Procedure, Parliament of
    Australia, Canberra, AU,
    www.aph.gov.au/About_Parliament/Senate/Powers_practice_n
    _procedures/Constitution/~/~/~/~/~/link.aspx?_id=6ED2CAE6
    1E7742A1B2C42F95D4C05252&_z=z, accessed March 8, 2014.

11 McLennan, G., *Understanding Our Christian Heritage,* vol. 1,
    Christian History Research Institute, Orange, NSW, Australia, 1989,
    p. 49.

12 Ibid., p. 51.

13 "Tom Roberts' Big Picture," Parliament House Art Collection,
    Parliament of Australia, Canberra, AU,
    www.aph.gov.au/Visit_Parliament/Parliament_House_Art_Co
    llection/Tom_Roberts_Big_Picture, accessed March 9, 2014.

14 McLennan, G., *Understanding Our Christian Heritage,* vol. 2,
    Christian History Research Institute, Orange, NSW, Australia, 1989,
    pp. 81–82.

15 "Recessional," 1897, notes by Mary Hamer, January 24, 2008, The
    Kipling Society, Essex, England.
    www.kiplingsociety.co.uk/rg_recess1.htm, accessed August. 12,
    2014.

16 https://www.abs.gov.au/articles/religious-affiliation-australia,
    accessed May 21, 2014.

Chapter 13
God in the Government of Canada

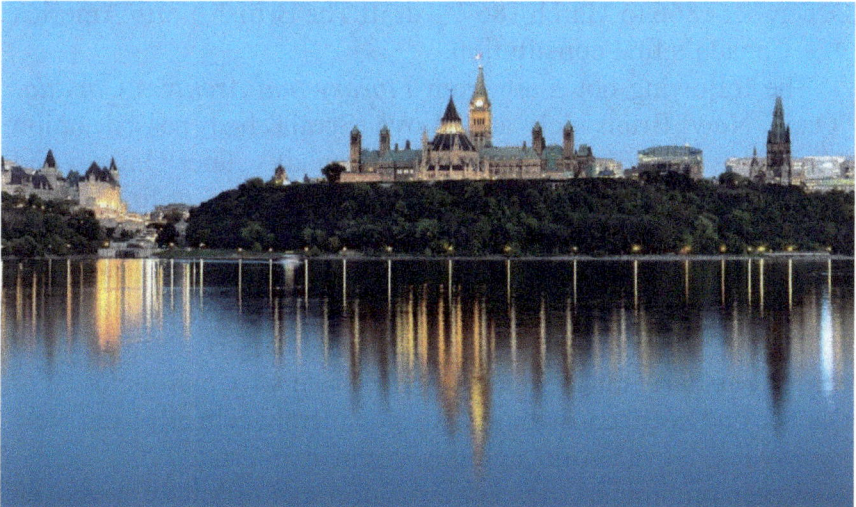

Songquan Deng/Shutterstock.com

THE PARLIAMENT BUILDINGS OF CANADA

So, Who IS This 'God' of Our Nation? This chapter and the science chapters show many reasons why students in Canada have the unalienable right to be taught "Why God is so highly recognized by their Government." He can provide wisdom, hope, food, grace, care, encouragement, understanding, and accurate knowledge for an abundant Life.

Our forefathers understood that God and His wise advice are integral parts of good government.

Note: Author's emphasis added by underlining.

Canada Becomes A Nation

The London Conference December 1866 – March 1867

The Fathers of Confederation met in London, England from December 1866 to March 1867 to draft The British North America Act, Canada's first constitution.

The following notes are from *Library and Archives Canada:* "Once New Brunswick and Nova Scotia had passed union resolutions in 1866 (the Province of Canada – later Ontario and Quebec – had already done so), it was time to meet to draft the text of the *British North America Act.* It was agreed that this meeting would take place in London. The Maritime delegates left for England on July 21, but for various reasons the Canadian delegation's arrival was delayed until late November. The conference was much smaller than those at Charlottetown or Québec had been, consisting of sixteen members in all (from New Brunswick, Nova Scotia, and the Province of Canada).

"After preliminary discussions, meetings officially began on December 4; they took place at the Westminster Palace Hotel in London. Business commenced with a thorough review of the Québec Resolutions to ensure that the wording of each was satisfactory. Despite Charles Tupper's promises to anti-union factions in Nova Scotia, he was unable to introduce amendments to the agreement at this time. Once the review was completed in late December, the "London Resolutions" were sent to the Colonial Office. Following the Christmas holiday, a committee of the delegates used the Resolutions to draft a proposed bill; copies were printed, and the delegates met with British officials in order to finalize the text.

"Choosing 'Canada' as the new country's name was relatively easy, as was the choice of 'Ontario' and 'Quebec' for the two halves of the Province of Canada. However, difficulties arose in choosing a designation. The delegates wished it to be a kingdom; the British feared that such a title would anger the United States, and denied the request. <u>An alternative, 'Dominion,' was suggested by Samuel Leonard Tilley, from a line in Psalm 72 of the Bible:</u>

"He shall have dominion also from sea to sea, and from the river unto the ends of the earth. " (This was adopted.)

"In addition to drafting the *British North America Act*, the Conference had to cope with the presence of an anti-union delegation from Nova Scotia, led by Joseph Howe, which was bent on overturning any union agreement. Charles Tupper was occupied in countering each submission Howe made to the Colonial Office and the two men conducted a debate through pamphlets and letters.

"The delegates had a completed text for the bill by the first week of February 1867. It was submitted to the Queen on February 11 and read in the House of Lords for the first time the following day. Proceedings were relatively uneventful: the bill passed through its first, second, and third readings in the House of Lords during the month of February. The three readings in the House of Commons were also swift, completed within two weeks with very little debate. The *British North America Act* received the Royal Assent on March 29, 1867.

"Once the Act was passed, the delegates returned home to prepare for union, which was scheduled to take place on July 1. Delegates from Nova Scotia and New Brunswick had to hold their final legislative sessions, in order to make last-minute changes to their constitutions. There also remained the task of selecting members for the new Cabinet and Senate.

"Social activities did not have the same prominence in London that they did at the other conferences, although some delegates did make excursions to other European countries, and visits to relatives and friends. For the most prominent of the delegates, there was also a royal audience. The major social event of the conference, however, was probably the marriage of John A. Macdonald (who became Canada's first Prime Minister) and Agnes Bernard on February 16, 1867." [1]

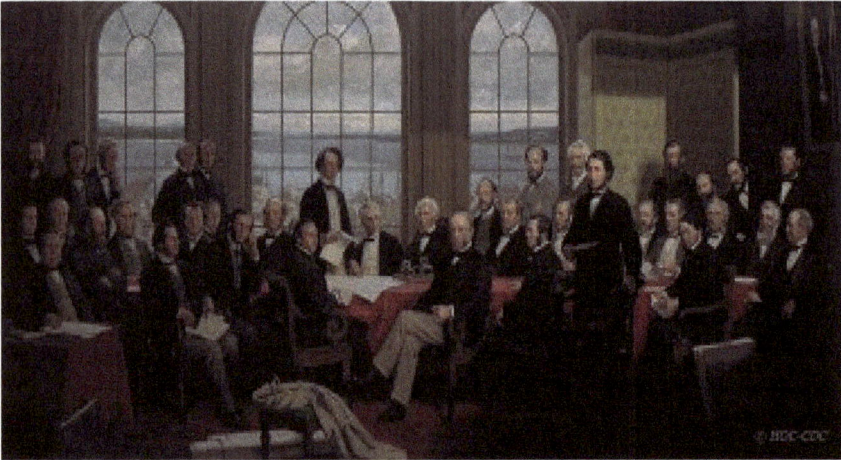

Reproduced with the permission of Rogers Communications Inc.

"THE FATHERS OF CONFEDERATION"
by Rex Woods, 1969.

"This reproduction of Rex Wood's 1967 oil painting depicts the delegates to the 1864 Quebec Conference at which the basis of the British North America Act was formulated and discussed. The painting is based on an 1883 canvas by Robert Harris that was destroyed in the 1916 House of Commons fire. Confederation Life commissioned Rex Woods to recreate the Harris painting and it was presented to the nation as a centennial gift." [2]

Canada's Fathers of Confederation:

Hewitt Bernard, secretary	Sir Alexander Campbell	Robert Barry Dickey
William Henry Steeves	Sir Adams George Archibald	Sir Charles Tupper
Edward Whelan	Sir Hector-Louis Langevin	John Hamilton Gray, N.B.

William Alexander Henry	Sir John Alexander Macdonald	William Henry Pope
Charles Fisher	Sir George-Etienne Cartier	William MacDougall
John Hamilton Gray, P.E.I.	Sir Étienne-Paschal Taché	Thomas D'Arcy McGee
Edward Palmer	George Brown	Andrew Archibald Macdonald
George Cole	Thomas Heath Haviland	Jonathan McCully
Sir Samuel Leonard Tilley	Sir Alexander Tilloch Galt	John Mercer Johnson
Sir Frederic B. T. Carter	Peter Mitchell	Robert Duncan Wilmot
Jean-Charles Chapais	James Cockburn	Sir William Pearce Howland
Sir Ambrose Shea	Sir Oliver Mowat	John William Ritchie
Edward Barron Chandler		

God is a part of a number of official documents and related content in the Government of Canada. Here are some key examples.

1. The Canadian Constitution (Excerpts)

"CONSTITUTION ACT, 1982

PART I

CANADIAN CHARTER OF RIGHTS AND FREEDOMS

__Whereas Canada is founded upon principles that recognize the supremacy of God and the rule of law:__ (Emphasis added)

Guarantee of Rights and Freedoms

1. The Canadian Charter of Rights and Freedoms guarantees the rights and freedoms set out in it subject only to such reasonable limits prescribed by law as can be demonstrably justified in a free and democratic society.

Fundamental Freedoms

2. Everyone has the following fundamental freedoms:
    a. freedom of conscience and religion;
    b. freedom of thought, belief, opinion and expression, including freedom of the press and other media of communication;
    c. freedom of peaceful assembly; and
    d. freedom of association.

Democratic Rights

3. Every citizen of Canada has the right to vote in an election of members of the House of Commons or of a legislative assembly and to be qualified for membership therein.

4. (1) No House of Commons and no legislative assembly shall continue for longer than five years from the date fixed for the return of the writs at a general election of its members.

(2) In time of real or apprehended war, invasion or insurrection, a House of Commons may be continued by Parliament and a legislative assembly may be continued by the legislature beyond five years if such continuation is not opposed by the votes of more than one-third of the members of the House of Commons or the legislative assembly, as the case may be." [3]

2. The Canadian Courts and Justice System
(Excerpts)

"Oaths of Allegiance Act
R.S.C., 1985, c. O-1
An Act respecting oaths of allegiance

SHORT TITLE

1. This Act may be cited as the *Oaths of Allegiance Act*. R.S., c. O-1, s-1.

OATH OF ALLEGIANCE

2. (1) Every person who, either of his own accord or in compliance with any lawful requirement made of the person, or in obedience to the directions of any Act or law in force in Canada, except the *Constitution Act, 1867* and the *Citizenship Act*, desires to take an oath of allegiance shall have administered and take the oath in the following form, and no other:

I, ..., do swear that I will be faithful and bear true allegiance to His Majesty King Charles the Third, King of Canada, His Heirs and Successors. <u>So help me God</u>. (Emphasis added.)

(2) Where there is a demise of the Crown, there shall be substituted in the oath of allegiance the name of the Sovereign for the time being.

R.S., c. O-1, s. 2; 1974-75-76, c. 108, s. 39.

SOLEMN AFFIRMATION

3. Every person allowed by law in civil cases to solemnly affirm instead of taking an oath shall be permitted to take a solemn affirmation of allegiance in the like terms, with such modifications as the circumstances require, as the oath of allegiance, and that affirmation, taken before the proper officer, shall in all cases be accepted from the person in lieu of the oath and has the like effect as the oath.

R.S., c. O-1, s. 5. [4]

3. The National Anthems

i. *The Royal* (Current official lyrics)

"<u>God</u> save our gracious King,
Long live our noble King,
   God save the King!
Send him victorious,
Happy and glorious,
Long to reign over us;
   God save the King!
 Thy choicest gifts in store
On him be pleased to pour;
Long may he reign;
May he defend our laws,
And ever give us cause
To sing with heart and voice,
   God save the King!" [5]

ii. **National Anthem** (excerpts as referenced)
The music for Canada's national anthem was written in 1880 by
Calixa Lavallée, known then as "Canada's national musician".
The music was commissioned to go with the French words of a
poem written by Judge Adolfe-Basile Routhie; the first perform-
ance was in Quebec City on June 24, 1880.

The unofficial English lyrics for Lavallée's music changed a
number of times until the words of a poem written by Judge
Robert Stanley Weir in 1908 were informally adopted as the
English version of the anthem. These words were altered slightly
until the first verse of his poem with the third-to-last line modified,
was officially proclaimed as Canada's anthem through the
National Anthem Act in 1980. The words are as follows:

O Canada! (English version)

O Canada! Our home and native land!
True patriot love in all our sons' command.
With glowing hearts we see thee rise,
The true north strong and free;
From far and wide, O Canada,
We stand on guard for thee.
God keep our land glorious and free!
O Canada, we stand on guard for thee,
O Canada, we stand on guard for thee.

Here is the balance of the original poem by Judge R. Stanley Weir
in 1908:
O Canada! Where pines and maples grow,
Great prairies spread and lordly rivers flow,
How dear to us thy broad domain, From
east to western sea!
Thou land of hope for all who toil!
Thou true north strong and free!
O Canada! O Canada!
O Canada, we stand on guard for thee,
O Canada, we stand on guard for thee.

O Canada! Beneath thy shining skies
May stalwart sons and gentle maidens rise;
To keep thee steadfast through the years
From east to western sea,
Our own beloved native land,
Our true north strong and free.
O Canada! O Canada!
O Canada, we stand on guard for thee,
O Canada, we stand on guard for thee

Ruler supreme, who hearest humble prayer,
Hold our Dominion in thy loving care.
Help us to find, O God, in thee
A lasting rich reward.
As waiting for the better day,
We ever stand on guard.
O Canada! O Canada!
O Canada, we stand on guard for thee.
O Canada, we stand on guard for thee!

iii. ***O Canada!*** (French version):
 O Canada! Terre de nos aïeux,
Ton front est ceint de fleurons glorieux!
Car ton bras sait porter l'épée,
Il sait porter la croix!
Ton histoire est une épopée
Des plus brillants exploits.
Et ta valeur, de foi trempée,
Protégera nos foyers et nos droits.
Protégera nos foyers et nos droits. [6]

4. Prime Ministers' and Their Party's Initial Throne Speeches (Excerpts)

The First Throne Speech was made to the Parliament of Canada on November 7, 1867, with the First Prime Minister, Sir John A. Macdonald in attendance. After the opening prayers, the Throne Speech was delivered by the First Governor General of Canada, His Excellency, The Right Honourable Charles Stanley: *".... I am happy to be able to congratulate you on the abundant harvest with which it has pleased Providence to bless you, and on the general prosperity of the Dominion. Your new nationality enters on its course backed by the moral support, the material aid, and the most ardent good wishes of the Mother Country. Within your own borders peace, security and prosperity prevail, and I fervently pray that your aspirations may be directed to such high and patriotic objects, and that you may be endowed with such a spirit of moderation and wisdom as will cause you to render the great work of Union which has been achieved, a blessing to yourselves and your posterity, and a fresh starting point in the moral, political and material advancement of the people of Canada."* [7]

Recent throne speeches at the opening of new Parliament Sessions, delivered to the Senate and the House of Commons by the Governor-General, have concluded with these words: *"May Divine Providence guide you in your deliberations and make you equal to the trust bestowed upon you."* [8]

5. Daily Proceedings in Parliament (Excerpts)

"Each of the three events in the Daily Proceedings—Prayers, Statements by Members, and Oral Questions—is covered separately in the Standing Orders.

i. Prayers

"Prior to the doors of the Chamber being opened to the public at the beginning of each sitting of the House, the Speaker takes the Chair and proceeds to read the prayer, after it has been determined that a quorum of 20 Members including the Chair Occupant is present, and before any business is considered. While the prayer is being read, the Speaker, the Members and the Table Officers all stand. The prayer is by custom read partly in French and partly in English. When the prayer is finished, the House pauses for a moment of silence for private thought and reflection. At the end of the moment of silence, the Speaker orders the doors opened. At this point, television coverage of the proceedings commences and the public may enter the galleries.

ii.   **Historical Perspective**

. . . "Until 1994, no major change to the form of the prayer was made aside from references to royalty. At that time, the House concurred in a report recommending a new form of prayer more reflective of the different religions embraced by Canadians. This prayer was read for the first time when the House met to open its proceedings on February 21, 1994:

"Almighty God, we give thanks for the great blessings which have been bestowed on Canada and its citizens, including the gifts of freedom, opportunity and peace that we enjoy. We pray for our Sovereign, Queen Elizabeth, and the Governor General. Guide us in our deliberations as Members of Parliament, and strengthen us in our awareness of our duties and responsibilities as Members. Grant us wisdom, knowledge, and understanding to preserve the blessings of this country for the benefit of all and to make good laws and wise decisions. Amen.

"When the House convenes on the first day of a new Parliament or on any day when the House is to elect a Speaker, the prayer is read after a Speaker has been elected. Indeed, at that time, the election of a Speaker must be the first order of business and has precedence over all other matters. Only after a Speaker has been elected, is the House properly constituted to conduct its business. After the House reconvenes following the election of the Speaker, the prayer is read before the House proceeds to the Senate to inform the Governor General of its choice." [9]

6. Canadian War Memorials

i.   The Tomb of the Unknown Soldier:

"The Tomb of the Unknown Soldier was created to honour the more than 116,000 Canadians who sacrificed their lives in the cause of peace and freedom. Furthermore, the Unknown Soldier represents all Canadians, whether they be navy, army, air force or merchant marine, who died or may die for their country in all conflicts – past, present, and future." [10]

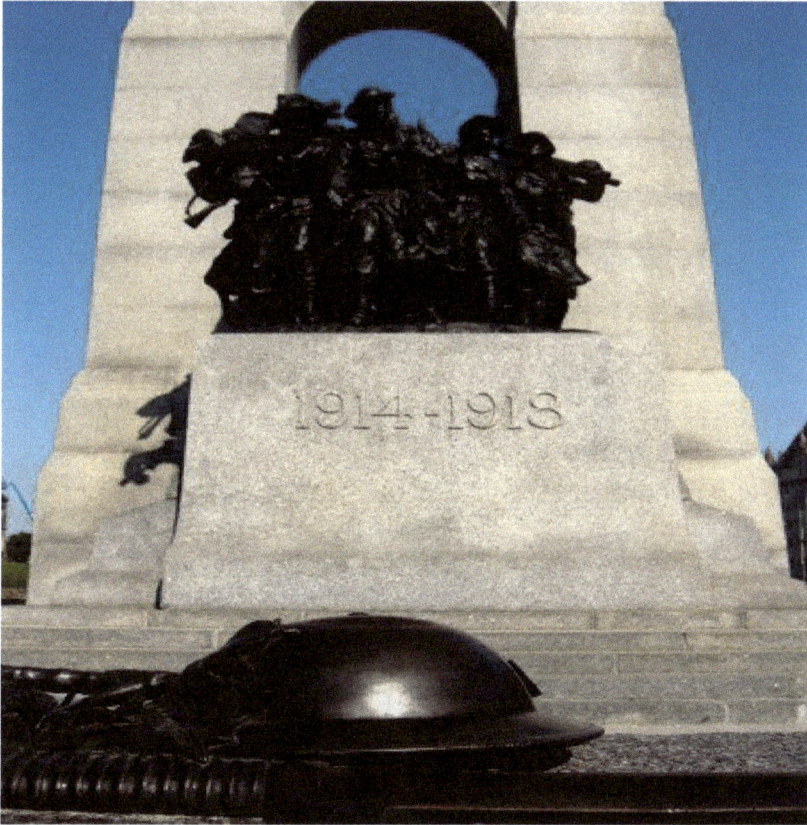

TOMB OF THE UNKNOWN SOLDIER
Ottawa, Ontario

ii.   **Victory Square Cenotaph, Vancouver:**

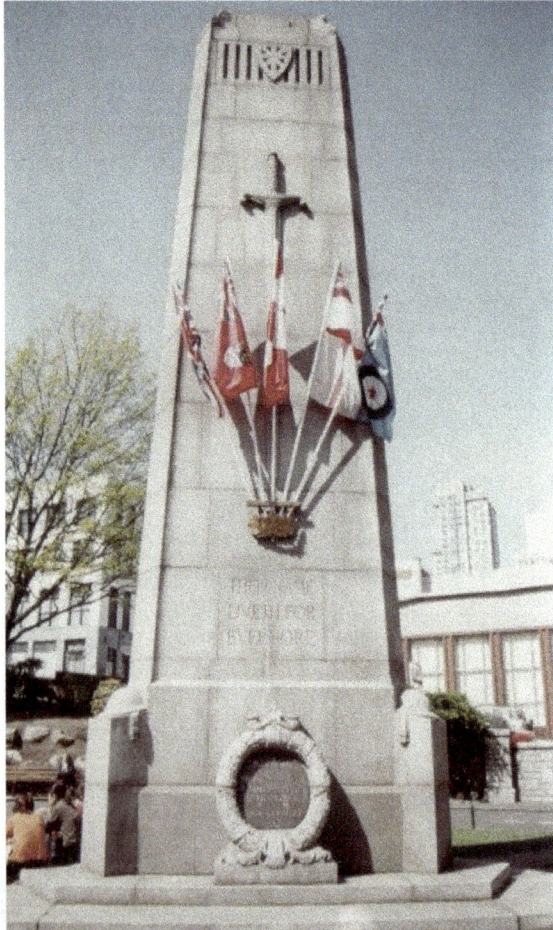

VICTORY SQUARE CENOTAPH
Vancouver, British Columbia [11]

This memorial bears the inscription "THEIR NAME LIVETH FOR EVERMORE."

The following excerpts are from a book, *Remembrance Day 1944: Service of the Armed Forces and Citizens, Vancouver, Canada,* written by Major J.S.Matthews and published by the City of Vancouver Archives:

"Those whose sacrifice this Cenotaph commemorates, were among the men who, at call of King and Country, left all that was dear, endured hardship, faced danger, and finally passed from the sight of men by the path of duty, giving their own lives that others might live in freedom. Let those who come after see to it that their names be not forgotten."

– Major the Reverend C.C. Owen

"The Cenotaph was unveiled by His Worship W.R. Owen, Mayor of Vancouver, in the presence of an assemblage of 25,000 persons, naval, military and civilian, and including The Old Contemptibles, 7th British Columbia, 29th Vancouver, 72nd Seaforth, 2nd Canadian Mounted Rifles, 47th New Westminster, and 102nd North British Columbia Battalions, C.E.F., and others, on Sunday, 27th of April, 1924. It was dedicated by Hon. Major the Reverend Cecil C. Owen, M.B.E., V.D., D.D., Chaplain of the 29th (Vancouver) Battalion, C.E.F., *"To the Glory of God, and in thankful remembrance of those who served King and Country overseas in the cause of truth, righteousness and freedom."*

"The 24th Psalm was read by Hon. Lt.-Col. the Rev. G.O. Fallis, C.B.E., E.D., D.D., of the Methodist Church, and the music included "O Canada" (Buchan); "O God, Our Help in Ages Past", "Lochaber No More" (bagpipes); "For All the Saints"; "Last Post" and "God Save the King." The first wreath, being the tribute of the Corporation and Citizens of Vancouver, was reverently placed by Mrs. W.R. Owen, wife of His Worship, the Mayor. J.S. Matthews, City Archives, City Hall, Vancouver, 1944." [12]

Hundreds of various memorials exist across Canada in cities and towns, honouring the brave souls who gave their lives in defense of Canadians, allies, and our precious democratic freedoms.

iii. **The poem, *In Flanders Fields*:**

"*In Flanders Fields* was first published in England's *Punch* magazine in December 1915. Within months, this poem came to symbolize the sacrifices of all who were fighting in the First World War. Today, the poem continues to be a part of Remembrance Day ceremonies in Canada and other countries throughout the world.

"The poem was written by a Canadian—John McCrae, a doctor and teacher, who served in both the South African War and the First World War.

"In Flanders Fields"

In Flanders fields the poppies blow
Between the crosses, row on row,
That mark our place; and in the sky
The larks, still bravely singing, fly
Scarce heard amid the guns below.

We are the Dead. Short days ago
We lived, felt dawn, saw sunset glow,
Loved and were loved, and now we lie,
In Flanders fields.

Take up our quarrel with the foe:
To you from failing hands we throw
The torch; be yours to hold it high.
If ye break faith with us who die
We shall not sleep, though poppies
grow in Flanders fields.

By Lieutenant-Colonel John McCrae" [13]

7. National Holidays that Honour God

Of the five national holidays in Canada for everyone, plus five additional holidays for federal employees and most other citizens, four are established specifically to honour God and His Son, Jesus. The first five national holidays include New Year's Day, Good Friday (Easter), Canada Day, Labour Day, and Christmas Day. The other five are Easter Monday, Victoria Day, Thanksgiving Day, Remembrance Day, and Boxing Day.

The first of the God-honouring four national holidays is <u>Good Friday</u>, which is established to honour the sacrificial death of Jesus Christ, the Son of God, who died to pay the penalty for the spiritual sins of all the people of the world who would recognize this as a gift of salvation and accept it.

The second is <u>Easter Monday</u>, which is established to honour the resurrection of Jesus from His dead state showing that God can give life to the dead physically as well as spiritually.   The third of the four is <u>Thanksgiving Day</u>, which is established to set aside a time to give special thanks to God for the harvest of the food He has made for us throughout the year plus all our other blessings.

The fourth is <u>Christmas Day</u>, which is established to honour the birth of <u>Jesus Christ, Son of God</u>. He was sent to teach us how to live a fulfilled and joyful life through loving our Creator and loving our neighbours as ourselves.

God is also honoured frequently on <u>Canada Day</u> and <u>Remembrance Day</u>, in national programs and events, and in leaders' prayers.

Each time that we sing our national anthem, "O Canada," at sports events and on other occasions, we are requesting "<u>God keep our land glorious and free.</u>"

8. Canadian Currencies that Honour God

The Canadian dollar has various abbreviations, names, and nicknames including CAD, C, Dollar, Buck, or Loonie; one hundred cents to the dollar.

The Godly connection with Canadian currency is that all the coins currently being changed from the image of Queen Elizabeth to the image of King Charles III and bear the inscription "D. G.

REGINA" which is short form of "DEI GRATIA REGINA", Latin for "BY GOD'S GRACE, KING." The Canadian dollar became the official currency for the Province of Canada (now Ontario and Quebec) in 1858.

After Confederation in 1867, the new Nation of Canada took control of the production of its currency. Coins are produced by the Royal Canadian Mint and the polymer bills are outsourced from the British American Bank Note Company.

Canada has an excellent credit rating and has been internationally admired for its astute fiscal management most of the time.

9. Public Buildings and Places that Honour God

When approaching the Peace Tower at the centre of Canada's Parliament Buildings, you can see foundational principles of Canadian government inscribed thereon: *He hath dominion from sea to sea* (Psalm 72, v.8) and *Give the king thy judgements, O God, and thy righteousness unto the king's son* (Psalm 72, v.1). Another verse inscribed on the Peace Tower is: *Where there is no vision, the people perish.* (Proverbs 29:18).

These indicate the type of wise government that Canada intended to provide. May our elected officials and government employees keep these concepts in mind.

Other Bible verses inscribed in Parliament's Memorial Chamber include Ephesians 6:13: *Wherefore take unto you the whole armour of God that ye may be able to withstand in the evil day, and having done all, to stand.*

Conclusion

The items and locations covered in this chapter are only a small sample of the honour, and respect shown by the federal government of Canada towards God and His involvement in governmental content. Much more information is available regarding His recognition and influence nationally, as well as all of His provincial and municipal involvement.

These inscriptions, and many others on public buildings, are there for the public to see and for guidance of our governments.

It is clear that God has been a significant help in the governance of Canada. His wisdom and guidance are always available and always beneficial to those of us who will consult Him by prayer and the study of His word, the Holy Bible.

Current Canadian Believers in God - Census 2021

Total – Religion	36,211,910
Buddhist	356,445
Christian, (not otherwise specified)	2,753,690
Anabaptist	144,045
Anglican	1,114,740
Baptist	435,590
Catholic	10,853,500
Christian Orthodox	622,650
Jehovah's Witness	136,990
Latter Day Saints	87,545
Lutheran	3,427,440
Methodist and Wesleyan (Holiness)	100,390
Pentecostal and other Charismatic	396,535
Presbyterian	301,140

Reformed	79,820
United Church	1,212,260
Other Christian and Christian-related traditions [5]	743,945
Hindu	827,675
Jewish	335,145
Muslim	1,774,660
Sikh	771,295
North American Indigenous spirituality [6]	79,860
Other religions and spiritual traditions	227,910
No religion and secular perspectives	12,528,655

Applications for Life:

1. What is the first sentence in the Canadian Constitution?

_____

_____

_____

2. How many fathers of Confederation does Canada have? ___

3. In the Oath of Allegiance for Canadian Courts and Justice Systems, point (1) the personal commitment is "So help me ___."

4. In the Canadian Royal National Anthem, the first sentence is,

_____

_____

_____

5. In the Canadian National Anthem, one request is, "_____
keep our land glorious and free!"

6. In the current Throne Speeches at the opening of Parliament
Sessions, what words does the Governor General conclude with?

_____

_____

_____

7. What are the words of the first sentence in the daily opening
prayer prior to each sitting of the Members of Parliament in the
House of Commons? _____

_____

_____

_____

8. What Godly symbol do most war memorials and soldiers'
graves bear, as also shown in in the war memorial poem, _In
Flanders Fields_? _____

9. Name four Canadian national holidays that honour God:

_____

_____

10. On Canadian currency coins, what is the meaning of the Latin
words and abbreviations, "D.G.REGINA" or "DEI GRATIA
REX"? _____

11. On the Peace Tower at the centre of Canada's Parliament Buildings, what are the words of the first inscription noted?

_____

12. From the last Canadian Census (2021), about what portion of Canadians state they are believers in God? _____

References and Notes:

[1] "The London Conference December 1866 – March 1867," Canadian Confederation, Library and Archives Canada, Ottawa, ON., www.collectionscanada.gc.ca/confederation/023001-2700e.html, accessed March 12, 2014.

[2] Reproduced with the permission of Rogers Communications Inc.

[3] "Constitution Act, 1982," Justice Laws, Government of Canada, www.laws-lois.justice.gc.ca/eng/CONST/page-15.html#docCont, accessed March 13, 2014.

[4] "Oaths of Allegiance Act," 1985, Justice Laws, Government of Canada, http://laws-lois.justice.gc.ca/eng/acts/O-1/page-1.html, accessed August 12, 2014.

[5] "National Anthem," The British Monarchy, London, England, www.royal.gov.uk/MonarchUK/Symbols/NationalAnthem.aspx, accessed July 9, 2014.

[6] "National Anthem: O Canada," Canadian Heritage, Government of Canada, Ottawa, ON, www.pch.gc.ca/eng/1359402373291/1359402467746, accessed July 10, 2014.

[7] "Thursday, 17th November, 1867," *Throne Speech*, Parliament of Canada, Ottawa, ON, www.parl.gc.ca/Parlinfo/Documents/ThroneSpeech/1-01e.pdf, accessed July 12, 2014.

[8] "Speeches from the Throne and Motions for Address in Reply," Parliament of Canada, Ottawa, ON,

www.parl.gc.ca/Parlinfo/compilations/parliament/ThroneSpee chaspx?Language=E, accessed November 28, 2016.

9 "Prayers, Daily Proceedings," *House of Commons Procedure and Practice*, 2nd edition, 2009, Parliament of Canada, Ottawa, ON, www.parl.gc.ca/procedure-booklivre/document.aspx?sbdid=af057bd0-f018-4fb4-bd754a2200729f05&sbpidx=2, accessed July 12, 2014.

10 Veterans Affairs Canada, *Tomb of the Unknown Soldier,* www.veterans.gc.ca/eng/remembrance/memorials/canada/tom b-unknown-soldier, accessed June 30, 2014.

11 War Monuments in Canada, *Vancouver: Victory Square Cenotaph,* www.cdli.ca/monuments/bc/victory.htm, accessed July 30, 2014.

12 Matthews, J. S., *Remembrance Day 1944: Service of the Armed Forces and Citizens, Vancouver, Canada,* City of Vancouver Archives, Vancouver, BC, Canada, 1944.

13 Veterans Affairs Canada, *In Flanders Fields,* www.veterans.gc.ca/eng/remembrance/history/first-worldwar/mccrae, accessed July 30, 2014.

14 https://www12.statscan.gc.ca/census-recensement/2021/dp-pd/prof/details/, accessed May 21, 2024

Chapter 14

The History of Why Nations Collapse Can Teach Us How to Protect Our Own Nation

"Those who cannot remember the past, are condemned to repeat it."   --- George Santayana, Philosopher

"Do not be overcome by evil but overcome evil with good."
                                        --- Romans 12:21

Why Nations Fall and What We Can Do To Save Ours

Every previous civilization in recorded history has eventually fallen. In recent historical memory alone examples include: China's traditional Confucian monarchy; the Turkish Ottoman Empire; the Royal House of Iran; and the mighty Soviet Empire. All collapsed with sudden totality after allowing major problems to accumulate.

While all these empires suffered from well-recognized structural, social, and economic flaws, few commentators and historians at the time, saw these challenges as threats to the very existence of these societies.

Most people — if they think about it at all — would view the possible decline and fall of modern Western civilization as a highly unlikely proposition. The modern state, with its supposed evolutionary adaptability, its representative democracy, ever-increasing technological development, and fluid market economies, would simply mold and adapt to any internal or external challenges it may face.

This was the alluring proposition of political philosopher Francis Fukuyama's hugely influential 1992 work, *The End of History and the Last Man.* He argued that the ascendancy of Western democracy — which followed the dissolution of the Soviet Union and the end of the Cold War — meant that human society had reached: "not just ... the passing of a particular period of post-war history, but the end of history as such: That is, the end-point of mankind's ideological evolution and the universalization of Western democracy as the final form of human government." [1]

Events since that time — the rise of radical Islam; the increasing fragmentation of society, family, and community; the increasing levels of depression, self-harm, and drug abuse in advanced western countries — indicate that this optimism was naïve at best.

Historians looking at the fall of civilizations often use as an example, the once-seemingly unassailable Roman Empire. With its ruthlessly efficient armies, its technological, economic, cultural, and social sophistication relative to its contemporary challengers, and its ability to adapt and absorb influences from other civilizations and cultures, it provides a rich example of the folly of seeming historical inevitability. With the invaluable benefit of 1500 years of hindsight, reasons for the decline of the Roman Empire are often listed as including:

— Economic upheavals and the over-reliance on slave labor;
— Geographical and territorial over-expansion and military over-spending;
— Government corruption and political instability;
— The increasing threat from migrating Germanic tribes from the North including the Visigoths, the Franks, Vandals, Burgundians, and Huns;
— Weakening of the Roman legions.

Francis Schaeffer in his book, *How Shall We Then Live* (in commenting on Edward Gibbon's seminal work, *The Decline and Fall of the Roman Empire*) marked five fatal attributes of Roman society in its slow but inevitable decay from about the third century AD:

"1. A mounting acceptance and approval of ostentatious displays of "show" and luxury (affluence);

2. Economic disparity creating a widening gap between the very rich and the very poor;

3. An excessive obsession with sexual gratification;

4. Decline of traditional and formalistic artistic conventions

236

*and their increasing substitution with outlandish and
absurdist styles betraying little originality and creativity.*
*5. An increasing toleration and desire to "live off the state
without any commensurate social obligations.* [2]

To many contemporary observers viewing -- with increasing
alarm -- current social and cultural trends of western society
entering the third decade of the third millennia AD, this catalogue
might sound depressingly familiar.

States don't fail overnight. The seeds of their destruction are
sown deep within their political institutions.

Is it culture, weather, disease such as the Black Death, even
Covid-19, or geography? What about war or some singular event
that re-writes history? In their book, *Why Nations Fail: The Origins of Power, Prosperity, and Poverty,* authors Daron Acemoglu
and James Robinson argue that man, not nature, sows the seeds of
his own destruction through political and economic institutions.

"Korea," they write, "to take just one example, is a remarkably
homogeneous nation, yet the people of North Korea are among the
poorest on Earth while their brothers and sisters in South Korea are
among the richest. The south forges a society that created
incentives, rewarded innovation, and allowed everyone to
participate in economic opportunities and religion…while the lack
of property rights by North Korea's economic institutions make it
almost impossible for people to own property; the state owns
everything, including nearly all land and capital. Agriculture is
organized via collective farms. People work for the ruling Korean
Workers' Party, not themselves, which destroys their incentive to
succeed." [3]

Commentator Bill Muehlenberg in the contemporary website,
Culture Watch, 7 July, 2006, observed:

"A lot of thought has gone into human mortality, and how we
can prolong life. Less thought has gone into the question of why
nations die. But nations, like people, do have a beginning, and do
have an end. Thus, it is worth looking at the questions of: how and
why do nations collapse?"

He goes on: "One common theme that emerges from those who
have thought carefully about the decline of nations is that often it
is the case that they collapse from within, instead of perishing from

without. Thus, Arnold Toynbee could rightly say, *'Civilizations die from suicide, not murder'."* [4] (Emphasis added).

Again quoting Muehlenberg, "British historian, Arnold Joseph Toynbee (1889-1975) is most famous for his magisterial, *A Study of History, 1934-1961.* In this 12-volume work, he examined the rise and fall of nations remarking: "*Of the twenty-two civilizations that have appeared in history, nineteen of them collapsed when they reached the moral state the United States is in now.*" [5] "Given that this observation is more than half a century old, how much more true could it be today?" [5A]

"Other historians have noted the seemingly suicidal tendencies of nations to self-destruct. American historian Will Durant (1885-1981) said: *'A great civilization is not conquered from without until it has destroyed itself within. The essential causes of Rome's decline lay in her people, her morals, her class struggle, her failing trade, her bureaucratic despotism, her stifling taxes, her consuming wars.'* [6] (Emphasis added.)

"In collaboration with his wife Ariel, Durant penned the monumental 11-volume series, *Story of Civilization,* between 1935–1975. The two also authored (among other works) the 1968 study*, The Lessons of History,* which encapsulated many of their observations on '**the tendency of nations to wither from within.**'

"Lord Macaulay (1800–1859), the English writer and historian, made a similar observation about the fate of democracies. He said that, *'the average age of the world's great democratic nations has been 200 years. Each has been through the following sequence:*
From bondage to spiritual faith.
From faith to great courage.
From courage to liberty.
From liberty to abundance.
From abundance to complacency.
From complacency to selfishness.
From selfishness to apathy.
From apathy to dependency.
And from dependency back again into bondage.'
(In a letter from Macaulay to a U.S. friend, 23 May, 1857)." [7]

Questions arising from this thoughtless progression from liberty and abundance to dependency and bondage include: Where are we now in this regular cycle? In other words, how far along are we at this moment on the road to this seemingly inexorable decay?

For those not just studying history as an academic field, but who also believe that the modern democratic state is the best model for maximizing human freedom, prosperity, and happiness, the more important question is: **Can we possibly escape this typical collapse?**

Are We Next?

Muehlenberg continues: "It is not hard to pinpoint where we are on Macaulay's timeline. The examples of corruption, selfishness, apathy, and decadence are all around. The easiest way to make this case is simply to open the daily newspaper. Recent newspaper headlines readily make the case. Consider just a few from the year 2006:

- *"Bibles banned (May 12, 2006)* *Bibles are being banned in hospitals and schools in order not to offend non-Christians.* (Fortunately, not everywhere, yet.)

- *"Pedophiles launch own political party (May 30, 2006)* *Pedophiles in the Netherlands are registering a political party to press for lowering the legal age of sexual relations from 16 to 12 and allow child porn and bestiality. The party, which plans to register tomorrow, says it eventually wants to get rid of any age limit on all sexual relations."* (Fortunately, it was not fully approved, at least not yet).

- *"Gay school guide: Teachers' manual rejects 'mum' and 'dad'. (June 4, 2006),* Victoria* (Australia) *schools are being advised to dump the words "mother" and "father" by a new teachers' manual that promotes the cause of same-sex parents."* (Fortunately, not everywhere, yet.)

In 2020, current news items included:
- *Rioters around the United States are supposedly protesting the violent and unwarranted death of a black criminal (who was apparently high on drugs) by white police officers in*

Minnesota. Rioters randomly destroyed private properties and attacked other civilians, including African Americans. Social media platforms then banned a number of conservative commentators from their sites for calling for a greater police presence and for describing the rioters as anarchists. Many of these arrested during the upheavals were improperly set free by local district attorneys who professed support for their "cause."

- *A recent Associated Press (AP) investigation revealed that more than 100 United Nations (UN) peacekeepers ran a child sex ring in Haiti over a 10-year period and none were ever jailed. The report further found that, during the previous 12 years, there had been almost 2000 allegations of sexual abuse and exploitation by peacekeepers and other UN personnel around the world that were never investigated.*

These examples show not only the usual catalogue of human vice, common enough in any age, but also the pervasive culture of conformity, cowardice, and moral compromise among our society's bulwark institutions. The preparedness of elected officials, bureaucrats, and even churches, to bow to the demands of the mob (*Ochlocracy* — tyranny of the mob, as the ancient Greeks described it) indicates a culture in steep decline.

An American sociologist and elected Senator once described such events as "Defining Deviancy Down," Democrat Daniel Patrick Moynihan (1927–2003) in an important 1993 essay — one that today would see him, ironically enough, evicted from his own party — decried the moral collapse in the West observing: "The amount of deviant behavior in American society has increased beyond the levels the community can afford to recognize, and that accordingly, we have been redefining deviancy so as to exempt much conduct previously stigmatized, and also quietly raising the 'normal' level in categories where behavior is now, (but would have been) abnormal by any earlier standard." [8] He asserted that **the saturation of evil in modern society was so complete that the only way to psychologically cope was to 'redefine' it.**

More than 2500 years ago the prophet Isaiah warned of the relabeling of such aberrant behaviors: **"Woe to those who call evil good and good evil, who put darkness for light and light for darkness,…..."** (Isaiah 5:20)

How Did We Come To This?

There is a long and a short answer to this vexing question. The long answer runs all the way from the 'Enlightenment' in 17th century Europe through Marxism and humanism, through the counter-culture of the 1960s, to the modern consumerist society. The short answer is: From about World War I (1914–1918) on, Western society has embarked on an historically devastating social experiment to see **what happens when we reject God.**

The normalization and celebration of gender dystopia; the epidemic of drug abuse and physical abuse in Western society; and record societal levels of depression and alienation, show that the results are now in. **For a society that so freely discarded the centuries-old virtues of duty, loyalty, hard work, and faith in God, the bill is now due. We, as a society, sowed the seeds, and are now reaping our own destruction.**

Muehlenberg continues: "We have tried to live as if there is no God, and we are now reaping the whirlwind.

"One modern prophet who shares this view, is the former Russian gulag prisoner, Alexander Solzhenitsyn.

"He exposed the industrial-scale slaughter and callous indifference to human life in the Soviet Union (USSR), the world's first post-God society in his [1973] seminal work, *The Gulag Archipelago.* He has written passionately and eloquently on this theme and the reasons for the grisly tragedy that has become human history since the start of the 20th century. His assessment is simple and yet profound: **"It is because we have forgotten God. That is why all this is happening to us."** (Emphasis added).

"This moral, ethical, and societal decline," Solzhenitsyn said, **"is directly connected to our widescale rejection of God."** [9]

Historian Will Durant offers this insight: "There is no significant example in history, before our time, of a society successfully maintaining moral life without the aid of religion." [10]

"Celebrated American-British poet and critic, T.S. Eliot (1888–1965), author of *The Hollow Men and The Waste Land* [11] essayed an important volume of articles in 1948 (*Notes Towards the Definition of Culture*) where he declared: **"If Christianity goes, the whole of our culture goes.** Then you must start painfully again, and you cannot put on a new culture ready-made. You must wait for the grass to grow to feed the sheep to give the wool out of which your new coat will be made. You must pass through centuries of barbarism. We should not live to see the new culture, nor would our great-great-great-grand-children: and if we did, not one of us would be happy in it." [12]

His thesis: "Throw out God and the work of 'civilization' becomes very difficult if not impossible. Again, Will Durant agrees: 'From barbarism to civilization requires a century; from civilization to barbarism needs but a day.'" [13]

Dangers of Darwinisms, or... How What We Believe, Determines Our Outcomes.

Let's look at a false and misleading concept from the mid-1800s that has done much harm to our society: Charles Darwin's opus, *On the Origin of Species by Natural Selection or the Preservation of Favoured Races in the Struggle for Life* (1859), created the myth that humans are hairless apes simply at the end of an unguided evolutionary ladder.

The Theory of Evolution (No God Needed) holds a large portion of the blame for our human decline into the decadence that leads to national collapse. Darwin's "Survival of the Fittest" attitude and disregard for our generous Creator and His wise guidance, has led to selfishness, crime, corruption, dishonesty, and a moral down-slide with its resulting STD's, fatherless children, depression and anxiety (even amongst the young), alcoholism, drug abuse, physical and sexual abuses, suicides, heartache and sadness.

This work, with its central thesis of "survival of the fittest" proved a rationale for some of the greatest atrocities of the late 19th and 20th centuries, from the desecration of tribal peoples who were considered to be anthropologically a lower level of subhuman, to lynching's in the Deep South, to Hitler's holocaust through his belief in a Master Race.

Australia, with its hunter-gatherer Aboriginal societies surviving thousands of years, was a subject for some of these dehumanizing Darwinian theories to be put into practice. Dr. Carl Wieland of Australia, documents [13A] one troubling episode that involved a German evolutionist, Amalie Dietrich (nicknamed the "Angel of Black Death") who came to large Australian pastoral properties in the 1860s asking the station-owners' permission to shoot indigenous inhabitants for specimen collections. This then involved removing the skin from dead aboriginals for stuffing and mounting for display in the Godeffroy Museum in Hamburg. Although evicted from at least one property for this barbarism, she shortly returned home with a number of "specimens." U.S. evolutionists were also strongly involved in this flourishing "industry" seeking to collect "specimens" of other "sub-humans." (See also Monaghan, David re: 'body-snatchers'.) [13B]

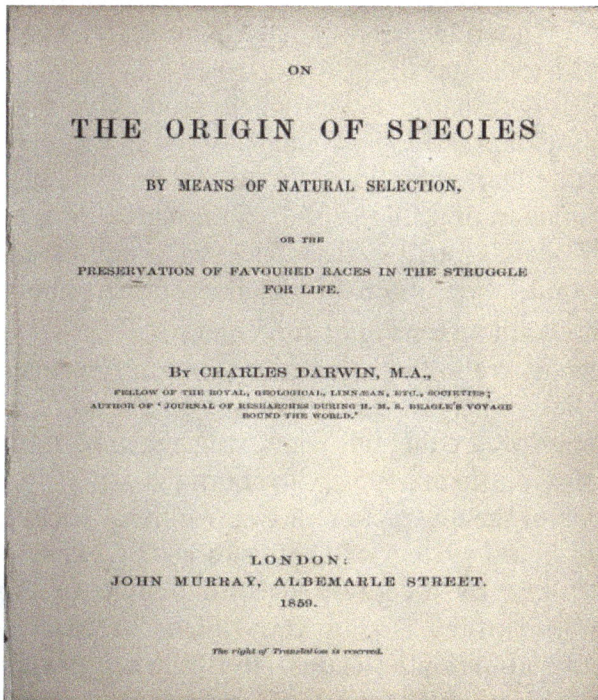

ON

THE ORIGIN OF SPECIES

BY MEANS OF NATURAL SELECTION,

OR THE

PRESERVATION OF FAVOURED RACES IN THE STRUGGLE
FOR LIFE.

By CHARLES DARWIN, M.A.,

FELLOW OF THE ROYAL, GEOLOGICAL, LINNÆAN, ETC., SOCIETIES;
AUTHOR OF 'JOURNAL OF RESEARCHES DURING H. M. S. BEAGLE'S VOYAGE
ROUND THE WORLD.'

LONDON:
JOHN MURRAY, ALBEMARLE STREET.
1859.

The right of Translation is reserved.

Wikimedia Commons

Along with museum curators from around the world, some of the top names in British science were involved in this large-scale, grave-robbing trade. These included anatomist Sir Richard Owen, anthropologist Sir Arthur Keith, and Charles Darwin himself. Darwin wrote asking for Tasmanian skulls at a time when only four full-blooded Tasmanian Aborigines were left alive, provided, he said, that his request would not "upset" their feelings. As with Dietrich, museums were not only interested in bones but also in fresh "skins" to provide interesting evolutionary displays when stuffed.

These 19th century eradicators and grave-robbers though were rank amateurs in comparison to the Darwinian adherents of the 20th century; the fascists of Nazi Germany and the Bolsheviks of the Soviet Union.

Adolf Hitler's belief in the superiority of the Aryan Master Race ("herrenvolk"), which he directly attributed to Darwinian theory, led to not just the industrial scale slaughter of Jews, Slavs, and gypsies ("Untermensch") but also eugenics, the killing of the disabled and handicapped.

Let's not forget that champion of "reproductive rights" in the United States, racist Margaret Sanger who, in the early 1920's, introduced this Darwinian ideology to America via abortion, the annual termination of millions of lives through killing the unborn. At the 1977 March for Life, Jesse Jackson asked, "What happens … to the moral fabric of a nation that accepts the aborting of the life of a baby without a pang of conscience?" [14]

If we humans are in fact, created by God in His image, and we now know how much superintelligent physical work with atoms plus the immense care that this takes, we have to believe that He is more than just a little unhappy with abortions.

How much of the destruction of His work will He tolerate?

The false belief system of evolution as the cause of life has been used since its inception to dull people to the societal benefits of Scripture. Using Darwinism to justify Nazism, Stalinism, the abortion holocaust, indifference to starvation in Africa, or the maltreatment of indigenous peoples, is all

against the wise Godly principles He has provided for our most civilized and enjoyable life.

In Europe, during what we now consider to be the barbaric 17th, 18th and 19th centuries, wars tragically cost the lives of several million people each century. But in our more enlightened, 20th century, it was not the more sophisticated weapons that created the untimely deaths of well over 70 million people, but the ideologies driving them to war, including Darwinian theory, Marxism, and the teachings of Friedrich Nietzsche ("God is dead").

Is There Anything That Can Be Done To Stop This Trend?

For those grieving at our torn society, weeping at the murder of innocents, at a society that celebrates the abuses of the powerful and strong against the weak and defenseless, is it now too late to repair what is broken?

As any engineer knows, the most important part of any building is its foundation. What is needed now more than ever is a rebuilding of the foundations of our society. As the Psalmist noted (Psalm 11:3): "If the foundations be destroyed, what can the righteous do?" For those willing to take up the tools, the job will not be easy, but for a better future, it must be done.

We as a society need to preserve and expand what is left of the good in our society and to resist those anarchic voices who would take it away from us. We must learn to speak, and to stand alone if need be, against the voices of dark destruction.

The first task is, as Santayana said, to learn from history in order to avoid repeating the major mistakes we encounter in history. It is not enough to recall the lessons of history. <u>We must be willing to act, to take a stand, to make a difference.</u> We cannot sit on the sidelines, shrinking from the fight, in a time of danger and threat. The greatest poet of the Renaissance, Dante Alighieri in his *Inferno,* wryly observed that: "The hottest level in hell is reserved for those who remain neutral in a moral crisis."

<u>At this crucial point in history, we all must get involved</u>. It is not enough just to talk about and define the problem, shake our heads sadly, and avoid the fray. <u>There are enemies of civilization who are all too involved in continuing to subtly destroy our nations from within.</u>

Muehlenberg states: "But what difference can one person make? Aren't the problems just too big? Legendary anthropologist Margaret Mead said otherwise: "Never doubt that a small group of thoughtful, committed citizens can change the world... indeed, it is the only thing that ever has." [15] Philosopher Edmund Burke also wrote: "Nobody makes a greater mistake than he, who did nothing, because he could only do a little." [16] In another context, radical Black Panther activist, Eldridge Cleaver, observed: "If you are not part of the solution, you are part of the problem." [17] Another Prophet, who was God in the flesh 2000 years ago, said: "You are the salt of the earth; you are the light of the world." (Matthew 5:13).

"So, what should we do, as believers? Often people debate as to whether we should seek personal revival or social reformation. This argument is often presented as an artificial either/or, yes/no, binary choice. But can I suggest that it is both/and. The need of the hour is to both get our own act together, and to seek to be a light in a dark world, to be a preserving salt ..."

It is less than a century since our Western democracies enjoyed "The Happy Days" of the 1950's. Personal honor and God-based principles were highly regarded and life was good. The U.S.A., the U.K., Australia, and Canada were all considered to be "Christian" nations. That was only 60 to 70 years ago.

To repeat, Lord Macaulay observed, "after the *faith, courage, liberty, and abundance*" of the 1950's, we headed into *"complacency, selfishness, apathy, dependency* (on the state)" to solve our problems, and now we are facing the *"bondage"* of excessive expenses, huge debts, and shrinking morals.

A major turning point happened in 1963 when atheist Madelyn Murray (O'Hair) and a few misguided friends were allowed to persuade the Supreme Court of the U.S.A. to outlaw prayers and other Godly benefits for American students. Other nations followed, and almost immediately there was a rampant rise in promiscuity, increased sexually transmitted diseases, many more fatherless children, anxiety, depression, drug abuse, increasing crime, and suicides. Many foolishly threw away the faith in our all-knowing Creator and Provider, along with the moral compass He provided for the benefit of all.

Understanding Our Enemies.

When I (Graham) trained as an officer during the Vietnam War, one of the "Principles of War" was *"Know Your Enemy."*

We must understand that there is an enemy of us all who works against us, but we can overcome evil with good.

Madelyn Murray O'Hair and friends were only one group whose work began to destroy America from within. **The religion of atheistic Humanism** expressed in their magazine, *The Humanist,* January-February, 1983: *"The battle for mankind's future must be waged and won in the public-school classroom by teachers who correctly perceive their roles as the proselytizers of a new faith... these teachers must embody the same selfless dedication as the most rabid fundamentalist preachers, for they will be ministers of another sort, utilizing the classroom instead of the pulpit to convey humanist values in whatever subject they teach, regardless of educational level - pre-school, day care or large state university. The classroom must and will become an arena of conflict between the old and the new - the rotting corpse of Christianity, together with all its adjacent evils and misery, and the new faith of humanism."* [18] WHAT A SEVERE PUBLIC THREAT THIS IS!!

One of the many unsubtle quotes of racist **Margaret Sanger, the founder and promoter of Planned Parenthood,** was*, "The most merciful thing that the large family does to one of its infant members is to kill it."* [19] Her work has led to the deaths of millions of unborn babies.

Also, the unscientific shortcomings of the evolutionary doctrine preached in our secular education institutions was summed up by an **open and honest evolutionist, Harvard Professor Richard Lewontin.** His words were, ***"We take the side of (materialist) science in spite of the patent absurdity of some of its constructs, ... Moreover, that materialism is absolute, for we cannot allow*** *a Divine Foot in the door.*" [11] (Emphasis added). (See pp. 88-89).

This blatant restriction is totally **anti-science.** It should be outlawed and exiled from the academic and scientific communities.

Teachers and professors have been fired for daring to suggest that there may be some intelligence in the way living entities are designed. This is obviously anti-science as it eliminates the foundational science principle of 'following the evidence wherever it leads'. As we have shown, it takes a superintelligent and caring entity (i.e., "God") to create and maintain living entities. Evolution, by definition, having no intelligence, is incapable of causing life.

What is not taught or spoken of enough, even in Christian churches, is the **understanding of the other supernatural entity known as Satan,** who subtly tempts unexpecting individuals and groups into making bad choices.

He can shrewdly make bad things look good (for a while). 'Try some of this special 'candy' (crystal meth). It will make you feel fantastic!' Then, with just one or two 'hits,' the unexpecting individual is trapped into such a horrific addiction that the rest of their usually short life is just a horrendous nightmare.

This is only one of Satan's thousands of subtle, destructive temptations that are gradually destroying the good life of individuals and our nations.

We have to wake up, understand, and resist this **"Public Enemy Number One!"**

Our nations are being destroyed from within, and that is where our healing must begin.

History from two to four millennia ago shows that collapsed nations were revived after they called out to the Creator for help.

Today, we have even the spokesman for the atheists of the world, none other than Dr. Richard Dawkins, telling the world through CBN News, "There are no Christians, as far as I know, blowing up buildings. I am not aware of any Christian suicide bombers. I am not aware of any major Christian denomination that believes the penalty for apostasy is death. I have mixed feelings about the decline of Christianity, in so far as *Christianity might be a bulwark against something worse."* [20]

It is the Christian community that provided the U.S.A., the U.K., Australia, and Canada with strong, functional and moral foundations years ago, and it will take a unifying effort by the current and future Christian community in these nations to lead the way in saving our nations from collapse. However, non-Christians have to participate as well if they want our nations to survive and improve.

To start, the restrengthening of the Christian community from its present weaknesses of timidity and retreating before threats, will come from a revitalized understanding of its potential influence-for-good through prayer and actions with God's help.

For examples, in the U.S.A., if the expression of "God Bless America," and in Canada's anthem, "God keep our land glorious and free," are treated as prayerful requests rather than arrogant demands, God may listen and respond more favorably. God also expects to receive more of the credit He deserves as our caring Creator and Provider.

Disrespecting God is a huge mistake as Old Testament history reveals time after time. His patience with us does have limits.

From the Dallas Times Herald, 10 May, 1980: "*The son of outspoken atheist Madalyn Murray O'Hair publicly apologized to Americans and God for his part in building 'the personal empire' of his mother: 'Looking back on the 33 years of life I wasted without faith and without God I pray that I may be able to correct just some of the wrong I have created,'* said William J. Murray of Houston in a letter to the editor of the Austin American Statesman.

" *'My crime was two-fold in that I was aware of the wrong of my actions at the time and continued them for the purpose of financial profit. I was continuing to practice the hateful anti-moral way of life I had learned from birth in an atheist home'.*

" *'The part I played as a teenager in removing prayer from public schools was criminal. I removed from our future generations that short time each day which should rightly be reserved for God. In as much as the suit to destroy the tradition of prayer in school was brought in my name. I feel gravely responsible for the resulting destruction of the moral fiber of our youth that it has caused' ".*

The main purposes of this book include firstly, to provide the basic science showing our personal creation and care by the superintelligent being known as "our Creator, the God of our focus nations;" and secondly, to reinforce the reasons for belief and appreciation for His essential provision of our food, our life, our best guidance, and wisdom; and thirdly, to provide a true science for the origin and cause of all Life.

We need to get back to knowing our Creator and benefitting from His wise advice. We need to stop our trivial pursuits and to realize that we are here for a great purpose.

An upgrade of attitude is essential to save our nations. *Freedom is not free!* Honorable lives have been personally given as payment. Let's not blow off our blessings by uncaring, ungodly, selfish neglect.

History shows us how nations decay from within.
Survival and Improvements Can Be Achieved
If We Choose to Care, Think, and Do What Is Right.

Recovery Must Come Through Us. Let's Do Something!
Here You Can Choose Your Commitments.

_____ My nation needs my help.

_____ I can share ideas from this book with friends.

_____ I can help my friends and neighbors.

_____ I can watch for people who are hurting and see if I can help.

_____ I can seek truth.

_____ I can get to know my Creator better.

_____ I can count my blessings.

_____ I can give God thanks for the many works He performs for me every second of every day.

_____ I can use the Ten Commandments as my life guide.

_____ I can see if my favorite school(s) would put the Ten Commandments somewhere visible.

_____ I can join a political party and try to be a good influence.

_____ I can regularly plan with friends to do something positive for our nation.

Applications for Life

1. How can I help my soul mate, parent, or child?

_____

_____

2. How can I get to know my Creator better each day?

_____

_____

3. What are the differences between North and South Korea and what have been some results since their 1953 war ended?

_____

_____

_____

4. Do you think Western civilization is collapsing? Why or why not?

_____

_____

_____

5. Will you commit to doing something positive for your nation or a neighbor every day? Even a prayer?

References and Notes:

[1] https://en.wikipedia.org/wiki/The_End_of_History_and_The_Last_Man

[2] Schaeffer, Francis, *How Should We Then Live – The Rise And Decline of Western Thought and Culture,* Crossway Books, Wheaton, IL, 1995, p. 227.

[3] Acemoglu, Daron and James A. Robinson, *Why Nations Fail: The Origin of Power, Prosperity, and Poverty,*(hardcover, Deckle Edge), Crown Business, New York, NY, 2012.

[4] https://billmuehlenberg.com/2006/07/07/when-nations-collapse/

(Muehlenberg cites the following authors to reference):

[5] https://en.wikipedia.org/wiki/Arnold_J._Toynbee
https://en.wikipedia.org/wiki/A_Study_of_History

[5A] https://billmuehlenberg.com/2019/01/17/on-the-decline-of-nations-and-their-possible-restoration/

[6] https://en.wikipedia.org/wiki/Will_Durant

[7] https://www.britannica.com/biography/Thomas-Babington-Macaulay-Baron-Macaulay

[8] https://en.wikipedia.org/wiki/Daniel_Patrick_Moynihan#cite_note-54

[9] Ericson, Edward E. Jr., *Solzhenitsyn – Voice from the Gulag,* Eternity, October 1985, pp. 23–24; https://en.wikipedia.org/wiki/Aleksandr_Solzhenitsyn

[10] https://www.sciencemeetsreligion.org/harmony.php

[11] https://en.wikipedia.org/wiki/T._S._Eliot

[12] https://en.wikipedia.org/wiki/The_Story_of_Civilization

[13] https://www.baltimoresun.com/maryland/carroll/opinion/cc-op-sprinkle-010420-20200104-opc3c76o4na47mtdtun4nvqw3y-story.html

[13A] https://creation.com/darwins-bodysnatchers-new-horrors Wieland, Carl, *Darwin's Body-Snatchers'*, Creation 12(3):21, June—August, 1990.

[13B] Monaghan, David, "The Body-Snatchers", *The Bulletin,* 12 November, 1991, pp. 30–38.

[14] https://www.gutenberg.org/files/1001/1001-h/1001-h.htm

[15] https://www.goalcast.com/2018/04/09/11-margaret-mead-quotes/

[16] https://en.wikipedia.org/wiki/Edmund_Burke

[17] https://en.wikipedia.org/wiki/Eldridge_Cleaver

[18] https://probe.org/education-and-new-age-humanism/

[19] https://www.lifenews.com/2013/03/11/10-eye-opening-quotes-from-planned-parenthood-founder-margaret-sanger/

[20] https://www1.cbn.com/cbnnews/us/2019/october/atheist-richard-dawkins-getting-rid-of-god-would-make-world-less-moral

THE HISTORY OF WHY NATIONS COLLAPSE CAN TEACH US HOW TO PROTECT OUR OWN NATION

Chapter 15
Choices and Consequences

In this book, we are looking at the nations of the U.S.A., the U.K., Australia, and Canada because it is historically noted that our Creator, God, provided a significant part of the foundational wisdom involved in the establishment and operation of these four nations. He continues to be a significant part, even though today a smaller proportion of our students, scientists, citizens, business leaders, and politicians are seeking His advice and guidance for their lives and work. By this choice, the good consequences for each are significantly diminished.

As every building is best served by a good, strong foundation, so it is with nations.

Through the decades, the beneficial, God-based operating philosophy of these four nations has attracted many immigrants from virtually all other countries of the world which do not have as attractive a governing system.

To what can we attribute the initial wisdom, strength, justice, integrity, stimulating atmosphere, attractiveness, and balanced growth of these four nations? – Certainly, when you look at the declarations, constitutions, and other founding documents and laws of these nations, it is easy to see the God-given principles adopted to guide our governments.

As with buildings, it is necessary that the whole structure is solidly *built, maintained, and repaired promptly when necessary*.

The Enemies Within (at least some that we know):

1)   As mentioned earlier, Public Enemy #1 (Satan himself) is the worst enemy for each of us and this includes our leaders. We have to see and resist his subtle temptations to make things look attractive or exciting now, but with damaging results in our future.

2)   Conspirators who know they cannot defeat our nations by attacking from outside, have developed ways to defeat our good systems from within our nations. For example, the conspiracy to

remove God's wisdom and other benefits from the lives of our students has been a devastating tool.

3) According to the Southern Poverty Law Center, there are 1430 hate and anti-government organizations in the USA now (2024).

4) Increasingly vulgar and violent movies, videos, games, and social media are playing a major role in degrading our culture.

5) Increased criminal activity including drug dealing, prostitution, sex-trafficking, fraud, scams, corruption, and greed all work against the good of our society.

6) Some conspirators have been allowed to interpret the "separation of church and state" ruling to mean the "separation of God and state." As explained, "the church" can be a building or a group of people who are Satanists, New Agers, Protestants, Catholics, Mormons, Muslims, Jehovah's Witnesses, and cults. They cannot <u>create</u> any living thing. *God is definitely not "the church" and they should not be confused as being the same.*

God is a significant and beneficial part of many churches, just as He is a significant and beneficial part of our governments.

Probably, the <u>worst choice</u> made by governments since 1960 was this:

In the early 1960s, a woman by the name of Madalyn Murray (O'Hair), an outspoken atheist with some atheist friends, influenced the U.S. Supreme Court to declare that prayer and Bible reading be banned from U.S. public schools.

The justice members did not realize how drastic the consequences for society would be from that terrible choice. Similar policies were adopted in the U.K., Australia, and Canada.

In the following years through today, there has been an appalling increase in drug and alcohol abuse, sexually transmitted diseases, births to unwed mothers (according to stats from the U.S. Department of Health and Human Services); violent behaviors and single parent families (according to the U.S. Department of Commerce, Census Bureau); and a major drop in academic achievement (according to the College Entrance Exam Board, New York).

The resulting emotional and physical devastations have led to further personal abuses, deep depressions, anxiety, and increased suicides. What a terrible choice that was in the early 1960s. The consequences have been absolutely abominable for our students, citizens, and nations.

Depending on the group of Christian students entering college or university, between 60% and 88% have their Christian belief bullied or persuaded out of them before they graduate. Then their future children lose out on God's guidance, wisdom, and benefits also.

What are the causes and how do we reverse this yearly downward trend?

At about the same time as Bible readings and prayers were removed from classrooms, the misleading and anti-science teaching of Darwinisms and evolution-only as the cause of life, began to be enforced in our secular schools and universities.

This was another terrible choice with widespread harmful consequences as it removed the teaching of understanding the individual care for each student by their Creator.

What a detrimental state for education to have descended into. *This enforced teaching of the lie of evolution as the origin and cause of Life is totally anti-science and anti-society.*

Fortunately, conscientious and brave scientists and educators are now choosing to back away from evolution as the cause of life, as much as they are allowed without losing their positions.

This is a beginning of restoration and recovery.

Nations today, as in past millennia, can deteriorate and collapse when they allow destructive choices to grow within them. They are like forms of national cancer and they are not new. We saw examples in the twentieth century and many more in the Old Testament and other history books as outlined in the previous chapter.

Michael Ruse, a devout Darwinist and author of *Darwin as Religion,*[1] documents the fact that "Darwinian thinking... has taken on the form and role of a religion; one in opposition to the world system, Christianity, from which in major respects it emerged."[2] This would be in opposition to the four God-based governing systems in the U.S.A., the U.K., Canada, and Australia, which we are focusing upon.

In Ruse's words, "Evolutionism or Darwinism is the *worldview* that Darwinists ushered in *to replace* the Creator-based world-view." He wrote, *"Evolutionary thinking became something more than a science hypothesis. It became a secular religion in opposition to Christianity. In the second half of the nineteenth century and the beginning of the twentieth century, Darwinian evolutionary thinking was gradually allowed to become an enforced education system countering and substituting for the Creator as the cause of life."* [3]

The result of rejecting Christianity and replacing it with Darwin in Ruse's own life was disastrous. He writes his con-clusion was, *"You are born. You live. Then you die. If you don't think so, then you should! We come from an eternity of oblivion. We return to an eternity of oblivion... In the end, you know truly that it doesn't mean a thing."* [4]

What a pathetic feeling to have at the end of one's life.

Ruse offers this view not only as his opinion, but as the supposed wisdom of past ages. He quotes celebrated Russian author Leo Tolstoy (1828-1910) who opined, *"everything we do and say ends up as stench and worms."* [5] However, Tolstoy later became a devout Christian and rejected this view. Ruse then quotes Harvard professor William James (1842-1910) who made the pronouncement, *"We are all such helpless failures in the last resort."* [6] He then jumps forward to the pessimist Albert Camus (1913-1960) who wrote, *"there is but one truly serious philo-sophical question, and that is suicide."* [7]

In the end, Ruse's attempt to determine if Darwinism is a religion that will satisfy mankind's craving for justice, love, purpose, and meaning concludes, in agreement with Darwinism, that the Darwinian world *"is a bleak world indeed."* [8]

What a sad Darwinist worldview for any individual.

On the other hand, Atomic Biology is not religion. It is pure science supported by research, experiment, experience, logic, common sense, and history. It gives us reasons to appreciate how much we are cared for by our reliable Creator, Sustainer, Main-tainer, Advisor, Friend, and Mentor.

What a great difference.

Since belief in evolution as the cause of life (knowing how brilliant and complex life is), requires immense faith, this makes evolution as much of a religion as any other belief requiring faith.

The huge difference is that the proponents of evolution have managed to arrange for teachers and professors to be their preachers of that humanistic religion and use our public schools, colleges, and universities as their churches. This should be illegal.

If we look at the troubled areas of our world today, we see the same problems with nations collapsing from within because they ignore the type of guiding advice and wisdom available in our manufacturer's manual, the Bible.

The four nations we are focusing on, started well but will not end well if upright principles of leaders and citizens are not practiced, taught, and cherished. Greed, immorality, and other poor choices will probably bring our downfall because they are destructive practices as history has proven. (See Chapter 14.) The signs are clearly evident.

This sounds like lecturing, and it is. A case can be made that the majority of us care about the well-being of our people and nations. As one wise person said, *"Real troubles come when good people do nothing."*

Good people, including and especially our students, are needed to **choose** to practice positive principles for good in their community and wisely help to repair what is deteriorating there and nationwide. It will take time and dedication to regain a more enjoyable society.

We, as individuals and nations, will enjoy life most by simply using the wisdom and advice of our Creator who cares so much and works so hard for each of us every second of every day. We can define wisdom as the practical application of beneficial knowledge, coupled with common sense and consideration for others. Part of this is defending ourselves and our society from further destruction by the crippling deceptive teaching of evolution as the cause of our life.

Understanding *temptation* is another huge part of wisdom. Temptations generally look attractive for a while, then turn around and give us troubles that can ruin the rest of our life.

Having the wisdom to *choose to turn temptations off at their beginning* can protect us from all kinds of trouble.

I am lecturing here because I care so much for our nations and good citizens. I hate to see anyone in unnecessary pain and suffering when wisdom and good choices are so readily available.

Regarding the best choices in science, the original concept of "following the evidence wherever it leads" is still the best path to choose. We believe the science of "Atomic Biology" will lead to the following benefits:
- an enjoyable appreciation of how much our Creator cares for us;
- a better understanding of our amazing bodies, minds, and gifts;
- happier attitudes;
- more wisdom for living;
- more nutritious foods;
- more beneficial and remedial diets;
- better medicines; and
- better health.

In the four nations we have focused on, we citizens are particularly blessed in many ways with plenty of food, shelter, clothing, comforts, health care, entertainment, etc. Our belief is that giving God "Thanks" at each mealtime and regularly counting our blessings is helpful in making our lives more enjoyable.

Hopefully, some principles and concepts in this book – and more so in the Bible – will help us and our governments to make more good choices resulting in at least some improved consequences nationwide.

There are some other theories regarding the cause of life that partially involve God and partially evolution, including Theistic Evolution, Evolutionary Creation, Progressive Creation, and variations thereof. However, we see attempts at compromise with each that cannot work in our opinion. 'Evolution,' as taught in our public education systems, is an unguided, non-intelligent, theoretical process, but creation and theism involve the most omniscient guide and creator in the whole world. How can we rationalize and accept an unguided/guided process as the cause of our life? It does not make sense and is misleading.

Our research revealed that every part of every cell in every living entity has to be superintelligently constructed with atoms. There are enormous numbers of significant decisions, choices and physical assembly works necessary throughout the construction of each cell part, cell, and living entity. Therefore, we believe that Atomic Biology is a more logical life science to explain the construction, sustenance, care, and maintenance for our lives.

Intelligent Design is another serious contender as the best scientific explanation for the cause of life but it stops short of the whole story. If you ask any architect, engineer, manufacturer, building contractor, or lad with a Lego set, you will get the same answer: a design does not **build** the project. **Superintelligent physical work** with atoms is essential to create each living entity.

After over three decades of research, we are proposing that **the God-honoring life science of "Atomic Biology" be considered seriously as the "best explanation" and best choice for explaining and teaching the origin and cause of life.**

Where it is accepted by various educators, it could be taught as the logical, evidence-based replacement for the currently taught but factually falsified theory of evolution.

We do not call this a "new" science because we believe our Creator has been using this since the beginning of life on Earth, along with the forces of gravity, electricity, magnetism, etc.

It would be very significant to find how many teachers, professors, and scientists actually doubt evolution is the real cause of life, if the threats and duress enforcing the teaching and proclamation of evolution-only, were made illegal, as they should be.

According to Bob Enyart's research, his *"RSR's 2014 List(s) of Scholars Doubting Darwin"* includes seven lists of scientists *"...who have gone out of their way to declare their doubt about Darwin...,"* plus websites showing *"...30,000 U.S. high school biology teachers who do not endorse Darwinism in class,"* plus *"100,000 college professors in the U.S. alone who, according to Harvard researchers, agree that intelligent design IS a serious scientific alternative to the Darwinian theory of evolution,"* plus *"570,000 medical doctors in the U.S., specialists in applied science, say God brought about or directly created humans."*

There is also Enyart's *"Honorable Mention: - 2.5 Million U.S. scientists and engineers believe in a personal God as reported by The New York Times in 1997..."* [9]

Dr. Francis S. Collins is a leading geneticist and was head of the Human Genome Project. In his book, *The Language of God: A Scientist Presents Evidence for Belief,*[10] he quotes Albert Einstein's "carefully chosen words" as saying, *"Science without religion is lame, religion without science is blind."*

Another quote from Dr. Collins, *"Science is not threatened by God; it is enhanced. God is not threatened by science; He made it all possible. So let us together seek to reclaim the solid ground of an intellectually and spiritually satisfying synthesis of all great truths. That ancient motherland of reason and worship was never in danger of crumbling. It never will be. It beckons all sincere seekers of truth to come and take up residence there. Answer that call. Abandon the battlements. Our hopes, joys, and the future of our world depend on it."* [11]

It is currently unfortunate that Dr. Collins tries to combine evolution and the Creator. Part of the problem is the six decades of teaching Darwinian evolution exclusively in our public schools. It includes a universal but unsubstantiated common ancestor and no God allowed.

In this book we expand substantially on the reasons why the Creator God of the Bible was formally and officially accepted into our governments at all levels in the four nations in our focus.

It is for these reasons, both scientific and historic, that **students especially, have the unalienable right to be taught "Why God Is So Highly Recognized by Their Governments."**

We are in no way suggesting this be construed as a particular "religion," other than its becoming a "belief as a truth." It can replace other current "beliefs" such as evolution, as the cause of life.

It is worthy of note that so many of the citizens in each of the four focus nations, claim to believe in God, according to census results noted at the end of our "God in Government" chapters.

If you think it through, you may agree that our Creator and Provider deserves our respect and appreciation for all the phenomenal, caring work He performs for each of us every second of every day.

This respect and appreciation is the reason for God's inclusion in our Governments in the first place.

Beyond His caring works for us is the hugely beneficial advice He gives to governments, teachers, students, business people, and all citizens who want it.

Applications for Life:

1. What type of foundation has proven to be best for nations in our world? _____

_____

2. After the foundation is well built, what type of work has been necessary to keep the nation functioning well? _____

_____

_____

3. What are some of the causes for troubles in the four nations we are discussing? _____

_____

_____

4. Who was one of the worst known conspirators? _____

_____

5.   What are four of the worst cultural problems according to government departments? _____

_____

_____

6.   What are four of the devastating personal problems that have resulted from these poor personal choices? _____

_____

_____

7.   What type of enforced teaching is totally anti-science and anti-society? _____

_____

_____

8.   What are some conscientious and brave scientists and educators now doing to resolve the above problems for students and other citizens? _____

_____

9.   What does Darwinist Michael Ruse consider Darwinism to be?

_____

10. Does this religion give him (or Prof. William James or Albert Camus whom Ruse quotes) satisfaction about life? _____

_____

_____

11. Some wise person said that "real troubles come _____

_____

12. Having the wisdom _____

_____

can protect us from all kinds of trouble.

13. What do you think about "counting your blessings" and saying "Thanks" to God for your food at meal-times? _____

_____

_____

14. Would you choose to believe that "Atomic Biology" as described in this book, provides a better explanation for the cause of life than the Theory of Evolution and why? _____

_____

_____

15. According to Bob Enyart's research, about how many scientists, biology teachers, college profs, medical doctors, and engineers in the U.S.A. indicate that they do not believe evolution is the cause of life? _____

References and Notes:

[1] Ruse, M., *Darwinism as Religion,* Oxford University Press, New York, NY, 2017.

[2] Ibid., p. ix.

[3] Ibid., p.5.

[4] Ruse, M., *A Meaning to Life,* Oxford University Press, New York, NY, 2019, p.1.

[5] Ibid., p.2.

[6] Ibid., p.3.

[7] Ibid., p.6.

[8] Ibid., pp.97, 133, 134.

[9] Enyart, Bob, *RSR's List of Scholars Doubting Darwin,* found at http://kgov.com/scientists-doubting-Darwin; accessed July 29, 2020.

[10] Collins, Francis S., *The Language of God,* Free Press division of Simon & Schuster, New York, NY, 2006, p.228.

[11] Ibid., pp.233-234.

Chapter 16
Next Steps Forward

Should We Teach Truth?

First of all, who, as a conscientious teacher or professor, wants to be known for teaching lies?

Problem #1 is that, at present, you don't always have a choice, and that hurts. Such is the case today. Truthful science, logic, observation, and common sense all provide solid evidence that the marvelous and beautiful living things around us are obviously designed and constructed by an intelligent being. However, most teachers and professors are forced by threat and intimidation to teach that there is no intelligence involved in the creation of living entities. This is **anti-science** and anti-society's well-being.

It is past time to stop the pretense that the God of our nations is not the Creator of Life, and to return to teaching Truth. Fortunately, according to Bob Enyart's findings as shown in the last chapter, tens of thousands of brave high school and university science instructors have found a way to indicate their disagreement with the theory of evolution.

Who among our education leaders will take a stand and work towards giving our Creator 100% of the credit for the origin and cause of life in all life science classes?

Reasons to upgrade:

1. False information is a very dull tool to be forced to use when designing a solution to any problem. Teaching true information is far better, more useful, and more honorable as well as more beneficial for students and society.

2. Falsehoods (lies) are misleading, deceptive, and costly road signs when traveling towards any goal. Accurate and truthful information is needed by our future leaders and problem-solvers.

3. The perpetrator of the falsehood, when discovered, is henceforth known as a liar and is humiliated. Honesty IS the best policy.

4. By what justification is teaching false information acceptable?

This newly discovered understanding of the superintelligence essential for building cell parts and living entities is not widely known, yet. However, it will be. Therefore, teachers and professors can keep this in mind and help the cause. We believe they will be more content with a legacy of teaching truth when it was verified rather than a legacy that says they continued to teach the lie of evolution as the origin and cause of Life.

Conclusion:

Here is a proposal to educators, as a sound and logical choice with significant and beneficial real-world consequences:

We propose a return to the trustworthy, intentional, and valuable basic scientific principle of "following the evidence wherever it leads and freely discussing it with students." This should never have been disallowed.

Substantial accumulated evidence verifies the essentiality of superintelligent physical works with atoms for building living cell parts, cells, and entities, including us. As a matter of scientific integrity, we recommend the introduction to the existing science curricula, the new evidence shown in this textbook for the best explanation of the origin and cause of all life.

This would also help students to understand "Why God Is So Highly Recognized by Their Government," now for scientific reasons.

If you would like to explore your possible participation in this project, you can contact us through our website at: www.atomicbiology.com

Our books can be customized by us to suit each interested group, e.g. adding or subtracting text, scriptures or messages.

Chapter 17
The Creator God Is In
All 50 State Constitutions

Every state constitution refers to the triune Creator God as in the US national government. Our creator God, from whom all our grown foods come, is either directly or indirectly written into all 50 state constitutions. The common expression "grateful to <u>Almighty God</u> for our freedom" refers to the belief that the source of our rights is not from government but rather from God. A good example is Maine's constitution that calls God the "Sovereign Ruler of the Universe." Delaware's says "Divine Goodness all men have, by nature, the rights of worshiping and serving <u>their Creator.</u>" The Virginia Bill of Rights refers to the duty that "we owe our Creator." The Washington State Constitution Preamble says "We, the People ...[are] grateful to the Supreme Ruler of the Universe." Teachers denied the right to critique Darwinism could simply teach their state's constitution. It could not be unconstitutional to teach the state's constitution! All 50 state constitutions acknowledge God, most as the creator, and the ACLU and the federal courts are wrong to deprive students of this knowledge. Below are the relevant sections compiled by Dr. Jerry Bergman.

Alabama 1901, Preamble: "We the people of the State of Alabama, invoking the favor and guidance of Almighty God, do ordain and establish the following Constitution."

Alaska 1956, Preamble: "We, the people of Alaska, grateful to God and to those who founded our nation and pioneered this great land, ..."

Arizona 1911, Preamble: "We, the people of the State of Arizona, grateful to Almighty God for our liberties, do ordain this Constitution."

Arkansas 1874, Preamble: "We, the people of the State of Arkansas, grateful to Almighty God for the privilege of choosing our own form of government; ...."

California 1879, Preamble: "We, the People of the State of California, grateful to Almighty God for our freedom, ..."

Colorado 1876, Preamble: "We, the people of Colorado, with profound reverence for the Supreme Ruler of the Universe, ... "

Connecticut 1818, Preamble: "The People of Connecticut, acknowledging with gratitude the good providence of God in permitting them to enjoy a free government, ..."

Delaware 1897, Preamble: "Through Divine Goodness, all men have, by nature, the rights of worshiping and serving their Creator according to the dictates of their consciences, ..."

Florida 1885, Preamble: "We, the people of the State of Florida, being grateful to Almighty God for our constitutional liberty, ... establish this Constitution."

Georgia 1777, Preamble: " .... we, the people of Georgia, relying upon protection and guidance of Almighty God, do ordain and establish this Constitution."

Hawaii 1959, Preamble: "We, the people of Hawaii, grateful for Divine Guidance ... establish this Constitution ....."

Idaho 1889, Preamble: "We, the people of the State of Idaho, grateful to Almighty God for our freedom, to secure its blessings ....."

Illinois 1870, Preamble: "We, the People of the State of Illinois, grateful to Almighty God for the civil, political and religious liberty which He hath so long permitted us to enjoy and seeking His blessing upon our endeavors ...."

Indiana 1851, Preamble: "We, the People of the State of Indiana, grateful to Almighty God for the free exercise of the right to choose our own form of government...."

Iowa 1857, Preamble: "We, the People of the State of Iowa, grateful to the Supreme Being for the blessings hitherto enjoyed, and feeling our dependence on Him for a continuation of these blessings, ..."

Kansas 1859, Preamble: "We, the people of Kansas, grateful to Almighty God for our civil and religious privileges ...establish this constitution ......"

Kentucky 1891, Preamble: "We, the people of the Commonwealth of Kentucky, grateful to Almighty God for the civil, political and religious liberties...."

Louisiana 1921, Preamble: "We, the people of Louisiana, grateful to Almighty God for the civil, political, economic, and religious liberties we enjoy.... establish this constitution."

Maine 1820, Preamble: "We, the people of Maine, ... acknowledging with grateful hearts the goodness of the Sovereign Ruler of the Universe in affording us an opportunity ... and imploring God's aid and direction....."

Maryland 1776, Preamble: We, the people of the State of Maryland, grateful to Almighty God for our civil and religious liberty...."

Massachusetts 1780, Preamble: We...the people of Massachusetts, acknowledging with grateful hearts, the goodness of the great Legislator of the Universe ... in the course of His Providence, an opportunity ...."

Michigan 1908, Preamble: "We, the people of the State of Michigan, grateful to Almighty God for the blessings of freedom, ... establish this constitution."

Minnesota, 1857, Preamble: "We, the people of the State of Minnesota, grateful to God for our civil and religious liberty, and desiring to perpetuate its blessings .... establish this constitution."

Mississippi 1890, Preamble: "We, the people of Mississippi in convention assembled, grateful to Almighty God, and invoking His blessing on our work, do ordain and establish this constitution."

Missouri 1845, Preamble: "We, the people of Missouri, with profound reverence for the Supreme Ruler of the Universe, and grateful for His goodness, do establish this constitution ...."

Montana 1889, Preamble: "We, the people of Montana, grateful to God for .....the blessings of liberty .... establish this constitution."

Nebraska 1875, Preamble: "We, the people, grateful to Almighty God for our freedom… establish ... the Constitution ....".

Nevada 1864, Preamble: We the people of the State of Nevada, grateful to Almighty God for our freedom, ... establish this constitution."

New Hampshire 1792, Part I. "Art. I. Sec. V. Every individual has a natural and unalienable right to worship God according to the dictates of his own conscience."

New Jersey 1844, Preamble: "We, the people of the State of New Jersey, grateful to Almighty God for civil and religious liberty which He hath so long permitted us to enjoy, and looking to Him for a blessing on our endeavors ... establish this constitution."

New Mexico 1911, Preamble: "We, the People of New Mexico, grateful to Almighty God for the blessings of liberty .....establish this constitution."

New York 1846, Preamble: "We, the people of the State of New York, grateful to Almighty God for our freedom, in order to secure its blessings, do establish this constitution."

North Carolina 1868, Preamble: "We the people of the State of North Carolina, grateful to Almighty God, the Sovereign Ruler of Nations, ... for our civil, political, and religious liberties, and acknowledging our dependence upon Him for the continuance of those blessings .... establish this Constitution.".

North Dakota 1889, Preamble: "We, the people of North Dakota, grateful to Almighty God for the blessings of civil and religious liberty, do ordain and establish this constitution."

Ohio 1852, Preamble: "We the people of the state of Ohio, grateful to Almighty God for our freedom, to secure its blessings and promote our common welfare, do establish this constitution."

Oklahoma 1907, Preamble: Invoking the guidance of Almighty God, in order to secure and perpetuate the blessing of liberty; .... establish this Constitution."

Oregon 1857, Article 1, Section 2: "All men shall be secure in the natural right to worship Almighty God according to the dictates of their own consciences."

Pennsylvania 1776, Preamble: We, the people of the Commonwealth of Pennsylvania, grateful to Almighty God for the blessings of civil and religious liberty, and humbly invoking His guidance ...."

Rhode Island 1842, Preamble: "We the People of the State of Rhode Island, grateful to Almighty God for the civil and religious liberty which He hath so long permitted us to enjoy, and looking to Him for a blessing upon our endeavors, ... establish this Constitution of government."

South Carolina, 1778, Preamble: "We, the people of the State of South Carolina, ... grateful to God for our liberties, do ordain and establish this Constitution ....."

South Dakota 1889, Preamble: "We, the people of South Dakota, grateful to Almighty God for our civil and religious liberties .... do ordain and establish this Constitution ...."

Tennessee 1796, Article 1, Section 3: "That all men have a natural and indefeasible right to worship Almighty God according to the dictates of their own conscience...."

Texas 1845, Preamble: "Humbly invoking the blessings of Almighty God, the People of the State of Texas, do ordain and establish this Constitution."

Utah 1896, Preamble: "Grateful to Almighty God for life and liberty, we, the people of Utah, ... establish this Constitution."

Vermont 1777, Chapter 1, Article 3: That all persons have a natural and unalienable right to worship almighty God, according to the dictates of their own consciences and understandings ...."

Virginia 1776, Bill of Rights, XVI : "Religion, or the duty which we owe to our Creator ..... can be directed only by Reason .... and that it is the mutual duty of all to practice Christian forbearance, love and charity towards each other."

Washington 1889, Preamble: "We, the People of the State of Washington, grateful to the Supreme Ruler of the Universe for our liberties, do ordain this Constitution."

West Virginia 1872, Preamble: "Since through Divine Providence we enjoy the blessings of civil, political and religious liberty, we, the people of West Virginia, in and through the provisions of this Constitution, reaffirm our faith in and constant reliance upon God ...."

Wisconsin 1848, Preamble: "We, the people of Wisconsin, grateful to Almighty God for our freedom, in order to secure its blessings, ... do establish this constitution."

Wyoming 1890, Preamble: "We, the people of the State of Wyoming, grateful to God for our civil, political, and religious liberties, ... establish this Constitution."

About the Authors

(Each has contributed to all chapters).

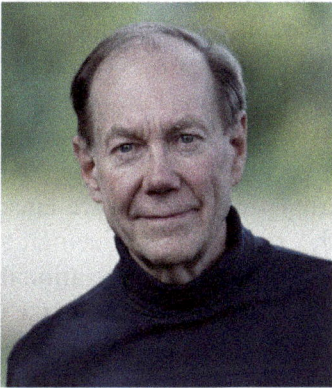

Dr. Jerry Bergman is a multi-award-winning professor and author. He has taught biology, biochemistry, anatomy, genetics, psychology, and other courses over 40 years at the University of Toledo, the Medical College of Ohio, Bowling Green State University, and other colleges. His prime academic degrees include two doctorates and his total of 1,026 college credits are equivalent to almost 20 master degrees. He is one of the most formally educated people in the world.

His 1400+ publications are in both scholarly and popular science journals. Dr. Bergman's work has been translated into 13 languages including French, German, Italian, Spanish, Danish, Polish, Czech, Chinese, Arabic, and Swedish. Books that include chapters he has authored are in over 1500 college libraries in 27 countries.

To date over 80,000 copies of the 60 books and monographs he has authored or co-authored are in print.

Beyond his classroom teaching, he has been an invited speaker at many colleges, universities, and church groups in America, Canada, Europe, the South Seas Islands, and Africa.

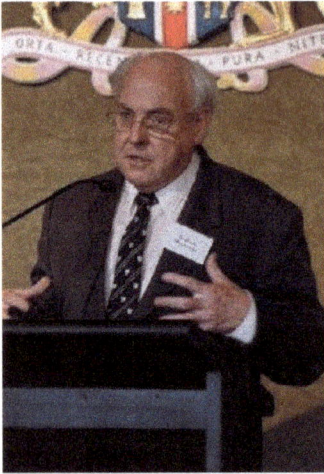
Ramon Williams/Worldwide Photos.

Dr. Graham McLennan is one of our co-authors and history advisors regarding the role of God in our Governments. His encouragement for this project of developing "atomic biology" as a new life science has been solid since 2011. Graham received his Degree in Dentistry from Sydney University, where he also became a Christian. He served as a Captain in the Australian Army; received the Defence Medal and the National Serviceman's Medal. Graham founded the National Alliance of Christian Leaders (NACL) with like-minded ministries in 1986.

Later, with his wife, Pam, they founded Christian History Research Institute in 1988 and later the www.chr.org.au website when the Bicentenary Celebrations occurred and he was on the executive of the National Gathering that surrounded the New Parliament House in prayer. More people turned out for this than the official opening by the Queen.

In 1993, Graham was an executive member of the Bicentennial of Christian Education, and in 2012 he initiated the National Christian Heritage Sunday celebrations. He received the Presidential Medal from the President of Vanuatu for "Services to the Nation."

He stood as a Senate candidate in 1984 and 1998 and supported others in local and state elections.

In addition to being a dental surgeon and tutor at the nearby University Dental School for many years, he also supervised dental students in Cambodia.

As convener of the NACL, Graham has been involved in helping initiate the Canberra Declaration, the Australian Christian Lobby, the National Day of Prayer and Fasting, and the Religious Freedom Institute (1990s). He is the founding Chairman of Rhema FM 103.5 and Orange Christian School. He is also a founding director of UCB's Vision FM and the Australian Christian Lobby and has served on many other national and international Christian boards and charities, as well as authoring Christian books and articles.

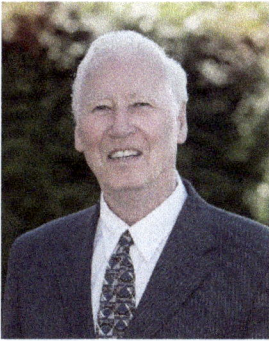

Thomas Rogers is an independent researcher, president of Reality Research and Development Inc., The Atomic Biology Institute, and other companies. He has studied at three universities and two specialty institutes. His work background includes engineering, research, construction, international manufacturing, and exploration.

The education and experiences in these fields helped him in 20 years of part-time and 17 years of full-time research into understanding the superintelligent physical works with atoms required to design, construct, sustain, maintain, and repair living entities, including us. Tom believes he has "done the time and paid the price" that might have earned him a PhD if performed under a different roof. However, the independence allowed him to think "outside-the-box" without biased restrictions and to stay focused on developing this verifiable God-based life science of "Atomic Biology" that goes a level deeper than molecular biology.

Tom has been a voluntary director of various community organizations, including the British Properties & Area Homeowners Association, the Greater Vancouver Apartment Owners Association, the West Vancouver – Howe Sound Social Credit Constituency Association, and he is a member of the Salvation Army and Calvary Baptist Church. He has memberships in the American Scientific Affiliation, the Canadian Scientific and Christian Affiliation, the Discovery Institute/Center for Science and Culture, the Creation Science Association of B.C., the Christian Scientific Society, and the American Association for the Advancement of Science.

Index: (See Glossary also on pp. xxi to xxix).

284

Credits and Permissions

The inclusion of any quotations, charts, figures, photographs, or other types of images in this book should not be considered as endorsements of the contents of this book by the copyright holders of those quotes or images.

Textbooks and Contact Information

With today's technology, our textbooks, booklets, summaries, courses, and talks can be **easily customized** to suit various groups or class settings like public schools, Christian schools, seminaries, church denominations, homeschools, colleges, and universities.

If You Would Like To Be Involved In Bringing God Back To Our Students:

The further development of this science for its numerous beneficial uses in addition to replacing Darwinisms as the taught cause of life, is an ongoing part of **"THE TRUTH FOR LIFE EDUCATION PROJECT"** by The Atomic Biology Institute.

We seek reputable scientists and citizens to become part of this historic new life science movement. If interested with comments, questions, or support for bringing God back to our classrooms, please contact us by the Contact Form at:

http://www.atomicbiology.com/contactus/